PRAISE FOR
*LIVING WELL WITH
MIGRAINE DISEASE AND HEADACHES*

"This book will be of great help and support to those suffering with Migraine and other chronic headaches. Teri's book goes a long way in helping the chronic headache sufferer understand that there are now effective methods of treating most headache problems. For those who wish to know more, the references in the various appendices are invaluable."

—Robert S. Kunkel, M.D., Cleveland Clinic Headache Center

"An upbeat, practical, and intelligent survey of our current understanding of Migraine and frequent headaches, written from the perspective of someone who is not a doctor or scientist but is a Migraine sufferer. Ms. Robert brings a balanced perspective to a field that suffers from both hype and oversimplification. A wonderful resource: timely, provocative, and funny."

—Elizabeth Loder, M.D.; director, Headache Management
Program, Spaulding Rehabilitation Program; assistant
professor of Medicine, Harvard Medical School

"A breath of fresh air for headache sufferers and their families, as well... Teri's book is more than a ray of hope: it is an annotated map for millions of sufferers who are wandering lost in a wilderness of pain and desperation."

—William B. Young, M.D., director, Inpatient Unit, Jefferson Headache Center, Thomas Jefferson University Hospital; associate professor of Neurology, Jefferson Medical College, Thomas Jefferson University, Philadelphia, Pennsylvania

"At the NHF, we know that informed patients are empowered patients who can work closely with their healthcare provider to improve their quality of life. With this book, you are well on your way to becoming this type of patient."

—Suzanne E. Simons, executive director, National Headache Foundation

"[O]ne of the most far-reaching books in educating the public about Migraine disease and headaches...Teri Robert's very detailed knowledge about Migraine disease certainly exceeds that of the vast majority of physicians...an invaluable guide and resource to all sufferers and their families...Her mission is focused, intense, illuminating and, ultimately, spectacularly empowering."

—John Claude Krusz, Ph.D., M.D., ANODYNE Headache and Pain Care

"This book is a wealth of knowledge, understanding, and compassion."

—Roger Cady, M.D., founder and director, Headache Care Center, Springfield, Missouri

LIVING WELL WITH

Migraine Disease and Headaches

LIVING WELL WITH
Migraine Disease and Headaches

What Your Doctor

Doesn't Tell You . . .

That You Need to Know

TERI ROBERT

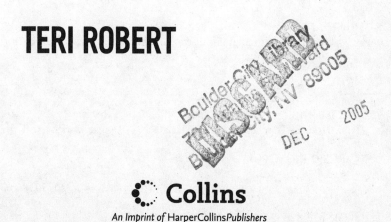

Collins

An Imprint of HarperCollins*Publishers*

HarperCollins books may be purchased for educational, business, or sales promotional use. For information please write: Special Markets Department, HarperCollins Publishers, 10 East 53rd Street, New York, NY 10022.

Designed by Joy O'Meara

Printed on acid-free paper

Library of Congress Cataloging-in-Publication Data

Robert, Teri.
    Living well with migraine disease and headaches : what your doctor doesn't tell you—that you need to know / Teri Robert.—1st ed.
       p. cm.
    Includes index.
    ISBN-10: 0–06–076685–9
    ISBN-13: 978-0-06-076685-6
  1. Migraine—Popular works. 2. Headache—Popular works. I. Title.

  RC392.R63   2005
  616.8'4912—dc22
                                 2005048456

05 06 07 08 09 WBC/QW 10 9 8 7 6 5 4 3 2 1

With affection, admiration, and hope,
I dedicate this book to all of you who live with
Migraine disease and headaches
and to those of you who are reading this book
because you care about someone else who does.
Keep learning, hoping, loving, and laughing.
Those are what will get us all through life in one piece.

Never forget:
You are not alone.
There is hope.

This book is also lovingly dedicated to those
who have lost their lives to Migraine disease, including

Sarah Crawford
Janice
and Abi Smith,

whose last request of me was to "keep educating people."

TOO SHORT

almost 22-years-old
almost, not quite
she visited a few times
then was gone
she needed
but gave more than she asked
then she was gone
she loved and laughed and cried
but then she was gone
was it with a whisper
or with a shout that she left?

In memory of Abi, from Teri Robert

CONTENTS

ACKNOWLEDGMENTS

You wouldn't be reading this book if I hadn't had the support of editor extraordinaire Sarah Durand, who has shown endless patience as I learned the process of writing a book and continually wanted to keep updating my manuscript rather than part with it. It's also her wisdom and foresight that sparked adding this book to the Living Well series. Two other people who made this book possible during its conception are my friend and colleague Mary Shomon, who had enough faith in me to recommend me for this project, and Carol Mann. Carol is Mary's agent, and she agreed to represent me on this book before we even met. At that first meeting, we took such joy in getting to know each other that we totally forgot about the contract we needed to sign! Thank you for believing in me, ladies.

Very special thanks go to my family and friends for their support and assistance. Hubby John has not only been supportive, but has fixed dinner for both of us most evenings while I was working. Our granddaughters Alexandra and Morgan inspire me because they're very young Migraineurs, and I naturally want their lives with Migraine disease to be easier than mine has been. Thanks also to my brother Ken, who has handled a few fire drills with my Web hosting company. True, that's his real-life job, but all I ever had to do was tell him there was a problem.

A huge thank-you must go to Michael John Coleman, who became a mentor of sorts when I started working in the area of Migraine disease. He was the first to recognize me as someone who was determined to make a difference and wasn't going to give up. He has shared his knowledge, insight, work, and friendship. As a fine-art photographer, he also wouldn't hear of anyone else taking my cover photo for this book! Michael, my eternal thanks to you and to everyone at MAGNUM.

There's another group of very special people I must thank—some quite brilliant doctors who work in the field of Migraine disease and headaches. Dr. William Young worked with me to gain control of my own Migraine disease and headaches, essentially returning control of my life to me. He also shared new research with me, answered all kinds of questions, and has encouraged my work every step of the way. His colleague, Dr. Stephen Silberstein, took time from his day to talk with me, answer questions, and take me on a whirlwind tour of the Jefferson Headache Center, introducing me to the staff. Dr. Fred Sheftell has, since the first time we spoke, treated me as a colleague and friend. He's never too busy to answer my questions. And what can I say about Dr. John Claude Krusz? We went from a simple telephone interview to his helping me answer questions for the "Ask the Clinician" section on my About.com site. I have learned more than I can tell you from working on this with him. He is always there, telling me I can do anything I set my mind to. To those doctors, add Dr. Jan Lewis Brandes, Dr. Steven Halpern, and Dr. Stewart Tepper. There are also the doctors whose research and work inspire me. Dr. Richard Lipton still leaves me in awe. Dr. Hans-Christoph Diener absolutely fascinated me when he was visiting during my first appointment at the Jefferson Headache Center. To all these doctors, plus those I didn't list, we all owe a great debt of gratitude. Thank you.

I also owe a great debt to my forum and chat hosts for my About.com site. They have managed the forums and chat room as well as I could have managed them myself, freeing me to write. They have also become my friends and part of my extended family. My forum members, too, are family. They love it when I'm there to talk with them but understand when I'm not. Not only do I offer them support, but they offer me support. As you read this book, you'll find a piece of advice that I had to include or never be allowed back in my forums because they love it so much. To all of you, I give my thanks and love.

For my friends who offered encouragement and listened to endless drafts of parts of this book, thanks are not enough. Cissy, Joan, Steven, Cliff, Nancy, Deb, Nicole, Stephen, Becky, you all deserve medals!

Finally, and perhaps most importantly, I have to acknowledge each and every person who suffers with Migraine disease and headaches as well as the people who love them. To this group, I add those who have lost their lives to Migraine disease and those who survive and mourn them. I send you thanks and blessings. It is my fondest wish that those of you who are suffering find effective treatment regimens soon and that those of you who are grieving find peace.

I feel as if I've just delivered an Academy Awards acceptance speech and as if I need to add a disclaimer here. I'm bound to have inadvertently left someone out of my thanks. Please know that I didn't mean to, and I do thank you!

FOREWORD

by Fred Sheftell, M.D.

First, I need to say how honored I am that Teri Robert has asked me to write the foreword for her important contribution to the field of headache and Migraine disease. There are many experts who would have been delighted to write the foreword, and I am truly proud that she asked me to do so.

Anyone who has been touched by headache or Migraine, be they sufferer, family, provider, employer, or friend, owes Teri Robert a debt of gratitude for her years of effort and advocacy on behalf of headache and Migraine sufferers and now her book. Reading through the pages, one can clearly see that this has been a labor of love and will serve as an invaluable resource for so many of us who work with and on behalf of headache and Migraine disease sufferers.

For twenty-five years I have heard the pain and anguish from so many whose lives have been devastated by headache disorders, Migraine disease and cluster headache in particular. Heaping insult onto injury are the stories of sufferers whose complaints have been minimized, doubted, and even dismissed! I have tried in my own small way to turn this around through my work with patients, teaching providers, as chairman of the World Headache Alliance for the past ten years, and as past president of the American Council for Headache Education. The National Headache Foundation has made monumental contributions to patient and physician education alike and honored Teri Robert last year at its annual fund-raiser for her work on behalf of sufferers.

Eighty percent of the patients referred to our center have chronic daily headache, and 80 percent are overusing a variety of over-the-counter (OTC) medications and prescription medications, mostly barbiturate-containing products (Fiorinal, Fioricet both with and without codeine, Esgic, and the like) and opiates (Vicodin, Lortab, Percocet, Percodan, and others). The problem of overuse (expertly described by Teri) is not confined to prescription medications. As one example, I can think of a man I saw in his late forties who prior to seeing us had been using eight ibuprofen tablets (Advil) per day for two years initially for episodic headache, which became daily over time. He began to notice black tarry stools and subsequently almost died secondary to developing three gastric ulcers that bled to the point where he went into hypovolemic shock, had virtually no blood pressure in the emergency room, and required three pints of blood. He was lucky—he lived. The story of Kellie as related by Teri and Kellie's mother did not have such an ending. This seventeen-year-old girl with her entire life in front of her died as a result of taking "just Tylenol" in quantities sufficient to cause acute liver and kidney failure! These stories are but a few of the tragedies that can occur with "just headache." (By the way, ever seen side effects and warnings on TV commercials for OTC products, the way you do for prescription products? I haven't.)

Teri's chosen "mission" has brought stories and questions from all over the globe to her Internet sites www.HelpForHeadaches.com and www.headaches.about.com, a true oasis for those in need. Not only can you get information and expert advice from Teri and her cadre of expert providers, but you can actually feel her smile and get an Internet hug! If you've never been to the sites, you will surely become a regular visitor after reading her book.

Teri begins by sharing her own story, which should be all too familiar to many of you with chronic headache or Migraine in terms of the pain itself, the impact on her life and on those who love her, the years of being doubted, and her search for help. She never gave up and tells her readers not to, either. Fortunately for so many of us, she turned her struggle in a positive direction by providing a road map of the pitfalls to be encountered on this road and by giving us accurate directions to find the right help and treatment for her fellow pilgrims. One of the many wonderful aspects of this book is her use of personal stories of sufferers who like herself have been willing to share their experience with us. The experience of my good friend Michael John Coleman as a child is another example. Michael John is another who on the basis of his experiences and struggles created an invaluable resource (MAGNUM), the National Migraine Association, for those who struggle with Migraine disease. These personal vignettes precede a discussion of what we need to know about a particular type of headache disorder, treatment, or empowerment technique, including getting around the many obstacles and detours thrown at us by "the system." That system includes "damaged" care (oh, excuse me, I meant "managed" care), limits or denials on treatments you require (by the way, my patients have never received letters from an HMO warning them that they may be overusing butalbital compounds or opiates, but as soon as they exceed nine triptan tablets per month . . .), emergency room interventions, hospitalization, getting your records, disability, and so forth.

The book is divided into five parts, with subchapters in each comprehensively covering the necessary topics from disease basics, treatment approaches and alternatives, support and empowerment, how to put it together, and finally appendixes providing the reader with easy-to-locate terms, resources, and references.

The most important nonpharmacological intervention is education. I'll never forget my patient who told me that when she questioned her previous doctor about the side effects of a particular medication and told him, "The *PDR* [*Physicians' Desk Reference*] says—" he slammed his hand on the table and said, "I hate when patients read the *PDR*!" I agree with my colleague Bill Young with respect to self-education. I've always disagreed with the statement that an educated patient is a dangerous patient, and like Dr. Young, I prefer patients who take an active role in their own treatment and enter a partnership-type relationship. The evidence suggests that those who come looking for the "magic bullet" and want something done to them to make it go way have an "external" locus of control, where someone or something outside of themselves will make it better, as opposed to those who have an "internal" locus of control, where they come in with the attitude "How can we work together to help my headaches?" This is a book for those who want to take that active role. All the tools, information, and resources you'll need are found in this wonderful book.

Just as Migraine is not "just a headache," this is not "just another headache book." It is a book of hope. If you are a sufferer, this book is a must; if you are touched by a sufferer, giving this book would be as good a gift as you will ever find.

Thank you, Teri Robert, for this book. And thanks to all of you who have struggled with us.

—Dr. Fred Sheftell, Director and Founder,
New England Center for Headache,
Stamford, Connecticut

INTRODUCTION

My Life with Migraine Disease and Headaches

The first time I remember having a Migraine attack was when I was six years old. At the time, I didn't realize what it was. There were these spots floating around in my vision that I couldn't see through. Then my head started hurting so badly that I began to cry. Crying just made it worse. It was a summer day, and the light coming through the window in my bedroom hurt my eyes, so I closed the curtains and buried my face in my pillow. I couldn't stay that way long because I needed to vomit. My father brought a large bowl from the kitchen so I didn't have to get up. Vividly, I remember him wiping my face with a cold cloth and rubbing my back gently until I fell asleep. My mother had these "headaches," too. At the age of six, I didn't really understand them, but I knew my mother would sometimes be in bed with her headaches for days. My parents have told me that the pediatrician said I was "high-strung" and had Migraines like my mother. All they could do was try to give me aspirin and hope I'd go to sleep.

There are many things about my childhood that I understand far better now that I know more about Migraine disease. My mother and an aunt who baby-sat my brother and me would frequently insist that I go outside in the summer to play. Playing outside on hot summer days often gave me "headaches," so I preferred to stay inside and read. During recess at school, I didn't want to jump rope or do other physical things in the sun. I wanted to sit quietly in a shady spot. That behavior brought criticism from my family and ridicule from other children. As a result, I was pretty much a lonely child with few friends. I did well academically and was far more comfortable with adults than with other children.

Through grade school and junior high school, my Migraines were infrequent. When I did get one at school, some teachers would insist that I stay in class but allow me to put my head down on my desk. They usually rethought that strategy once I'd vomited in their classrooms. Other teachers would send me to the nurse's office. Depending on the nurse, I'd either be told to lie down there or my parents would be called to come get me. One junior high school physical education teacher accused me of faking to get out of her class. My father went to school and took care of that problem very quickly.

By the time I was in high school, the other kids were old enough that not all of them were so insensitive to someone who was ill. I was able to make more friends. Since my Migraines weren't very frequent, I was actually able to have some social life. My parents had also gotten to the point of letting me stay home from school, without questions, when I didn't feel well.

College in the early 1970s was a different situation entirely. Some doctors still thought Migraines were psychological or a "woman's thing" and were very patronizing. Triptans were still years in the future, so doctors either told me to take aspirin or, if I was lucky, wrote me a prescription for pain medication. I spent my first semester of college at a large university, and the professors (for the most part) didn't consider a "headache" reason enough to miss a class session, let alone an exam. More than once, I was accused of having partied too much the night before or of using drugs. At the end of that semester, I transferred to a smaller branch of the university, where I found the professors to be far more understanding and accommodating. It helped that the campus nurse was also a Migraineur. I could go to the infirmary when I needed to, and she'd help me. She not only took care of me, she'd send an assistant to take notes to the professors of any classes I was missing, telling them where I was. One professor, who didn't allow exams to be made up, actually sent his graduate assistant to the infirmary with the exam I was missing to allow me to take the exam orally since I couldn't read it with my Migraine. Such were the advantages of a smaller college and, I'm told, of having a high grade-point average.

When I was in my early twenties, my Migraines gradually became more frequent and more severe. My family doctor sent me to an ENT (ear, nose, and throat specialist). That brilliant man (yeah, right) examined me, then said, "Congratulations. You're an intellectual. You have Migraines." I didn't know it at the time, but that was the beginning of twenty years of going from doctor to doctor seeking help. I don't know what it was. Maybe it was his tone of voice, but I knew this doctor was not going to be of any help to me. My family doctor, when he got the report from the ENT, wasn't any help, either. He just told me that "lots of women have Migraines. All you can do is take your pain pills and live with them." So that's what I did, for then.

A few years later, I changed family doctors. I kept insisting there had to be something that could be done about my "Migraine headaches." He sent me to see a neurologist. The neurologist did his thing with the light in my eyes, checking my reflexes, and that was it. Then he said, "Okay. You have Migraine headaches. What do you want me to do about it?" Duh! I wanted him to do something to help me! His advice? "Have a baby." He said that having a baby sometimes helped. Yes, well, I was divorced and living alone. That wasn't going to happen anytime soon. At my insistence, my family doctor sent me to a different neurologist. He ordered X-rays of my head and neck, and I thought maybe I'd found a doctor who was going to help me. So much for that thought. When I went back to see him after the X-rays, he said, "They're Migraines. That's what everyone else has told you. Now that we've done the X-rays, you can quit worrying. They're just headaches." When I said they weren't like other headaches I sometimes had, he said, "No, Migraines are worse, but if you'd quit worrying about them, you wouldn't have so many. Have you considered seeing a psychiatrist?" I replied, "I'm sick, not crazy." He answered, "I didn't say you were crazy, but you bring a lot of your headaches on yourself worrying about them and other things." I wasn't as gutsy then as I am now, so I didn't fire him on the spot, but I never went back, either.

Over the years, I'd had to go to the emergency room for my Migraines, but not often. When I was twenty-eight, I had to go to the ER with one, and they asked if I had a history of high blood pressure. I didn't, but there is a history of it in my family. My blood pressure was high that day, but they said it could have been high because of the Migraine and advised me to follow up with my family doctor. As it happened, I had just changed family doctors to go to a new one whose office was across the street from where I worked. When I went to follow up with him, I was diagnosed with hypertension. At the same appointment, he introduced me to a new Migraine medication, Midrin. Midrin worked better than other medications I'd tried, but it never worked as well for me as it does for some Migraineurs. This doctor, too, was very patronizing, simply patting me on the shoulder and telling me I'd just have to "put up with" the pain the Midrin didn't relieve.

When I was in my early thirties, my Migraines were wreaking havoc with my life. I was newly married, with two newly acquired teenage sons, and had gone back to college full-time. Unfortunately, I was also having severe Migraines, sometimes two or three times a week. I couldn't care for my family, go to class, or even function for days at a time. Yet another local neurologist was a total waste of time and money, so our family doctor referred me to a neurologist a ninety-minute drive away. My first thought when I met this doctor was that he had to be someone's grandfather. It was more than his age; he looked gentle and kind, and he really looked at me when we talked. More important, it seemed that he was actually listening to me! Then came some of the most precious words I had ever heard: "If you're willing to be patient and work with me, you don't have to live like this." That statement actually brought tears to my eyes. For the first time, this doctor explained to me that there were medications that, when taken on a daily basis, could actually help *prevent* my Migraines! Nobody had ever told me that before. Thus, he was the first doctor to tell me about Migraine preventives and prescribe one for me. After almost a year of periodic appointments and medication adjustments, the medication was keeping my Migraines pretty much tamed. It seemed miraculous, but I was having only about six or eight Migraines a year!

This blissful state of existence lasted for several years. Although this doctor had helped me gain control of my Migraines, he hadn't taught me anything about them, even that Migraine is a disease. Thus, I was still very ignorant of even the basics and thought this wonderful reduction in my attacks would last forever. Well, forever turned out to be several years, but that was hardly forever. By the time I was in my early forties, the frequency of my Migraines was increasing again. Unfortunately, my grandfatherly neurologist had retired. I'd already been to and fired every neurologist in my hometown, so my primary care doctor referred me to another neurologist a ninety-minute drive away. She was also supposed to be a Migraine specialist.

This neurologist's office and way of doing things was different from any I'd ever seen before. I lasted through two appointments with this one. Both times, I saw a nurse practitioner first. Then a doctor breezed in for less than five minutes and wouldn't even let me get an uninterrupted sentence out of my mouth, let alone answer any questions. A new preventive medication was prescribed at the first appointment. At the second, I was told to continue it, with no changes, even though I was making no progress.

My Migraines didn't get better. They got worse. I called the neurologist's office about a month later and was told to just keep taking my medication and keep my appointment. There was another problem, too. The preventive medication was causing serious side effects. Getting desperate, I called the neurologist's office a month before my appointment was scheduled. Again, they told me to keep taking the medication and keep my appointment. This was the beginning of the end of my being a doormat. I told the receptionist to cancel my appointment and prepare a copy of my records for me to pick up. She replied that she couldn't give me my records but would be glad to forward them to another doctor. I informed her that she not only *could* give me a copy of my records but was *required by law* to do so and told her what day I'd be there to pick them up. The day I picked up my records, the neurologist came out of her office to ask what the problem was. I looked her square in the eye and said, "You are. You're incompetent, and you are *so* fired." While she was struggling to pick her chin up off the floor, I left.

At this point, you may wonder what happened to make such a change in my attitude. I'll tell you: I'd started educating myself. It had become obvious to me that there wasn't a doctor within one hundred miles of my home who was going to help me, so I was going to have to find a way to help myself.

Where I live, you don't find much medical information in the libraries, so I hit the Internet. About.com is a network of nearly five hundred topic sites. Each individual site is written and managed by a "Guide" with expertise in and a passion for his or her topic. The About.com Diabetes site had already been very helpful to me because the Guide who ran it had already done the research for me. I could go there, read her articles, find links to other sites with good information, and get support from other people in similar situations with their diabetes. Given that experience, I decided to see if About.com had a site for Migraines but was disappointed to see that it didn't. It didn't take me long to discover that the Internet has vast amounts of information about headaches and Migraine. Unfortunately, not all of it is accurate, and it can be difficult to figure out what's accurate and what's not. By chance (or maybe not), I went back to the About.com health sites to look around and saw a "Be a Guide" link. There, I discovered that About.com was looking for someone to build a site on their network about headaches and Migraine. It struck me that I couldn't be the only person having so much trouble, so I applied for the position, and I got it. As I researched to write for the site, I was shocked at how much there was to know about Migraines that nobody had ever told me, including the fact that there were actually doctors who specialized in treating headaches and Migraine. I started the forums for the site and began to meet other Migraineurs. A couple of them told me about the Jefferson Headache Center in Philadelphia. They were patients there and had gotten much better since beginning their treatment at "the Jefferson."

Having just fired the last neurologist, I made an appointment with my primary doctor. I needed his help to taper off the preventive medication I was on. While I was there, I talked to him about a referral to the Jefferson. Yes, Philadelphia is an eight-hour drive away, and I had discovered other specialists closer to home, but I'd been fighting this situation so long that I wanted to go to the Jefferson because I'd talked to people who were being treated successfully there. My doctor agreed and called them for an appointment for me. We were shocked to find that the first available appointment was nine months away! He agreed to prescribe triptans and help me until that appointment.

Finally, the day of my appointment arrived. I'd been told that the appointment would take between five and six hours. A health history and a short psychological evaluation form had been sent to me to complete in advance and bring with me. When I arrived, I was impressed by the atmosphere of the reception area and waiting room. There were no overhead fluorescent lights in the waiting room. The lighting was subtle, but bright enough to read and complete forms. The room was quiet, and there were signs posted asking people not to wear fragrance to their appointments. (Fragrances are Migraine triggers for many people.) The receptionist took my insurance information and gave me a lengthy psychological survey to complete. Shortly, a nurse asked me to accompany her. She went over my medical history and family medical history in detail, entering the information into a computer as we went. She also asked a multitude of questions about my Migraines and symptoms and got the standard information of height, weight, blood pressure, and so on. She then showed me to a place where I could finish the forms I'd been given and wait to see the psychiatrist. I'll admit to you, as I did to the doctors that day, that I had a chip on my shoulder about seeing a psychiatrist. I think the poor man had been warned that I wasn't answering any of his questions until he answered mine. I suspect he'd met such resistance before, as he was very kind about it and not a bit patronizing. I actually had one question: Since Migraine is a neurological disease, just why did I have to see a psychiatrist as part of my treatment? He told me it was a fair question and that the answer had two parts:

1. Since there is a link between Migraine disease and clinical depression, part of the psychiatrist's job is to assess patients to see if they're also experiencing clinical depression. If they are, he needs to see that they're being treated and that the treatment is appropriate and working. He may have suggestions for changes. If the patient has untreated depression, he needs to make treatment suggestions.
2. Since any chronic illness requires good coping skills and strategies, it's also his job to assess each patient's coping skills and strategies to see if they're adequate of if they need assistance in developing and/or improving them.

Ahhhhhhhh. That was a perfectly acceptable explanation. It made a great deal of sense, in fact. Treat the whole patient, the whole disease, not just the symptoms. He told me that the short evaluation form I'd brought back with me had already been reviewed and showed no problems. He'd have the longer one reviewed and let me know if he saw any reason for another appointment, but he doubted that would be the case. At the end of our session, he told me that he didn't see a reason for him to treat me, but he would be available for me if I ever wanted to see him.

The last part of that first appointment was to see my new neurologist, who specializes in treating headaches and Migraine. Dr. William Young had reviewed the information the nurse had entered into the computer and the psychiatrist's evaluation. I had taken fairly recent MRI (magnetic resonance imaging) films with me, so he put them on the film viewer. He conducted a neurological examination. He checked reflexes, tested strength on both sides of my body, looked at my eyes, listened to the arteries in my neck with his stethoscope, performed various checks for balance and coordination, and more. Then, he showed me that my MRI films showed no problems. They displayed good, clear blood vessels, which he explained he looks for when he's considering prescribing triptan medications such as Imitrex, Zomig, and the like. We then discussed both my family and personal Migraine history and my general health, and we reviewed my Migraine diary.

Then it was time to discuss a treatment plan. He said that he'd prefer to change some of the medications I was already taking for other conditions before adding medications. Since blood pressure medications and antidepressants are often effective Migraine preventives, that's where we started. He changed the medications I was taking for those conditions and explained that it would take some time to know if they were going to work. He also prescribed both a triptan medication to actually stop a Migraine in progress and a pain medication so I wouldn't use either of them more than two days a week. Since I was having Migraines four or five days a week, he instructed me to take the triptan two days a week and the pain medication two other days a week, if necessary. That was to avoid rebound headaches, which can be caused by taking medications too often.

At my next appointment, there was no progress to report. Since neither the preventives prescribed by other doctors nor the preventives Dr. Young had prescribed were working, he suggested that we should rule out a physical condition that could cause headaches and trigger Migraines. Since it could be diagnosed only by doing a spinal tap, we scheduled it, and it showed that I did indeed have that condition.

The spinal tap and resulting treatment turned out to be a major turning point for me. Simply by taking a medication twice a day, that condition can be controlled. Right away, approximately 50 percent of my Migraines were gone—the 50 percent for which I hadn't been able to identify triggers and that had been accompanied by tinnitus (a ringing, hissing, or buzzing sound in my ears). Three months later, my Migraine diary showed a marked improvement, but there was room for more. I kept returning every three months and we'd fine-tune my regimen a bit more. After a couple of years working with Dr. Young, with the medications adjusted and dietary supplements added to my regimen, I was getting pain-free periods of up to forty-five days between Migraines. Then, to add insult to injury, I developed chronic daily tension headaches. Dr. Young wasn't too surprised. I'd had shoulder surgery, and my movement was significantly impaired. The glaucoma I'd had for several years had progressed to the point of requiring last-resort surgery. The bottom line was that if the surgery didn't work, I'd be blind in a couple of years. We added a medication to my preventive regimen to address the daily headaches. Not only did it stop the tension headaches, but it increased the length of time between my Migraines. That's where I am now with my preventive regimen. Knowing my Migraine triggers helps. They're disrupted or lack of sleep, skipping meals, changes in weather, and crying. As I write this, I haven't had a Migraine for over two months. It took time and patience to get to this point, but Migraine disease is no longer controlling my life, I'm controlling it. The last time I thanked Dr. Young, he reminded me that we did it as a team.

My treatment for when I do get a Migraine isn't as simple as it used to be. Imitrex was wonderful. With it, I seldom lost more than two hours to a Migraine, often less. Unfortunately, I was diagnosed with coronary artery disease about a year ago, and that meant the end of my being able to take medications such as Imitrex. Triptans work, at least in part, through the action they have to constrict blood vessels (make them smaller). Unfortunately, triptans don't totally confine that action to the blood vessels surrounding the brain, so they're not recommended for anyone with heart disease. So my "miracle" is no longer an option for me. We've tried various "pain pills" and anti-inflammatories, but I might as well be swallowing breath mints for all the good they do. I had to make one trip to the emergency room because I had a severe Migraine and no medications that would touch it. When I arrived at the ER, the triage nurse checked my blood pressure. It was considerably higher than would be safe for anyone, let alone a patient whose chart indicates coronary artery disease. I've never been treated as quickly as I was that evening. That Migraine attack showed Dr. Young and me that we had a secondary problem. While I might be able to get through the pain since my Migraines are so infrequent, the elevated blood pressure is dangerous. Ultimately, since I have so few Migraines, he wrote a prescription that allows me to do IM (intramuscular) injections of the same medication they used in the emergency room. Having it at home, I inject it into my thigh as soon as the pain begins, and that keeps the pain and my blood pressure from getting out of control. I also have both oral and injectable antinausea medication to use as necessary. Handling Migraine attacks in this way is possible only because I have so few of them now.

In addition to my other treatments, I was recently asked to try a new over-the-counter Migraine remedy, GelStat Migraine. It's a gel containing feverfew and ginger, and it's used by squirting it under the tongue, holding it there for sixty seconds, then swallowing it. You repeat it in five minutes. Not for an instant did I think that "stuff" was going to do a thing for my Migraines. I fully anticipated it was going to taste absolutely horrid and be a total waste of time. But I figured I'd try it, then tell them it was worthless and be done with it. The first time I tried it, I had the very beginning of head pain that I'm still not sure was Migraine or a tension headache. Whatever it was, it stopped. "Okay, that was just a fluke," I thought. The second time I took it, it did nothing. The third time, I took it at the beginning of a Migraine aura, two doses as described. After thirty minutes, still feeling a Migraine in early stages, I took two more doses. The Migraine never progressed any further. GelStat Migraine doesn't work for me every time. On the other hand, given how limited my treatment options are, I'm grateful that it works part of the time.

Throughout the years that I've struggled with Migraine disease, there have been times when the emotions I experience during a Migraine attack would bring me to my knees, ready to surrender. The strength of the emotions is pretty much proportional to the severity of the Migraine attack. Although I've never felt suicidal, there have been times, especially when I was alone, when I pretty much wanted to die. The only times I've ever experienced panic attacks have been during my worst Migraine attacks. I've now learned that there's a physical explanation for this, and we'll take a look at it in this book.

My family has been absolutely stellar through all of this. My husband has driven me to and from Philadelphia and sat in the hotel room, waiting, while I went for my appointments. He sat in the waiting room while I had the spinal tap. When I have a Migraine, he'll quietly ask if I need anything, but for the most part he leaves me alone because he knows that's what I want. Our sons are grown with families of their own. I had a Migraine at a time when one of them was visiting with his children. The girls were probably about three and five years old at the time. It's hard to ask young children to be quiet, so I retreated to the recliner in my home office. Periodically, I'd see two little heads peek around the corner to look at "Granny." Then they'd quietly tiptoe away.

Friends? Well, let's say that illness can show you the difference between friends and acquaintances. An acquaintance is there for you when all is well and you're fun to be with. Friends are always there. My experience is probably much like that of most people with headaches and Migraine disease. I have lots of acquaintances and a few good friends. The people who participate in the forums on my Web sites often thank me for my support. Believe me, it works both ways. I count on those forums and the people there for support, too. We're all in this together. Overall, with the family and friends I have, I am blessed.

PART ONE

Headache and Migraine Disease Basics

1

What Are Headaches and Migraine Disease?

Before we delve more deeply into the details of Migraine disease and headaches, it will help to have some background information about how many people are affected by Migraine disease and headaches, and some basics on the different kinds of head pain disorders will give us a base to build upon.

Not only is headache painful, but headache disorders are also disabling. Worldwide, according to the World Health Organization, Migraine alone is 19th among all causes of years lived with disability. Headache disorders impose recognizable burden on sufferers, including sometimes substantial personal suffering, impaired quality of life and financial cost. Repeated headache attacks, and often the constant fear of the next one, damage family life, social life, and employment. For example, social activity and work capacity are reduced in almost all Migraine

sufferers and in 60% of TTH (tension-type head-ache) sufferers.
        —From the World Health Organization

Migraineurs required 3.8 bed rest days for men and 5.6 days for women each year, resulting in a total of 112 million bedridden days. Migraine costs American employers about $13 billion a year because of missed workdays and impaired work function; close to $8 billion was directly due to missed workdays. Patients of both sexes aged 30 to 49 years incurred higher indirect costs compared with younger or older employed patients. Annual direct medical costs for migraine care were about $1 billion, and about $100 was spent per diagnosed patient. Physician office visits accounted for about 60% of all costs; in contrast, emergency department visits contributed less than 1% of the direct costs.
        —Hu XH et al.
    "Burden of migraine in the United States: disability and economic costs."
        Archives of Internal Medicine.

The Human and Economic Impact of Migraine Disease and Headaches

The preceding statistics are startling for more than one reason. Not only do they show how much time Migraineurs lose to Migraine, but when carefully examined, the $100 spent per diagnosed patient makes it clear that most Migraineurs aren't getting the care we need and deserve. Think about it. That $100 will barely cover one office visit. That substantiates something we already know—Migraine is a very underdiagnosed and undertreated disease.

Here is more information about how many people are affected by Migraine disease and headaches and the economic impact:

- Tension-type headaches and Migraine disease are the two most common head pain disorders.
- Of the people who consult their primary care physician for head pain, 94 percent have Migraine disease or Migraine-type headache.
- More than 90 percent of patients who go to their doctor for what they think are sinus headaches actually have Migraine disease.
- Migraine disease affects 18 percent of women and 6–8 percent of men. Those percentages convert to the following statistics:
  - *Nearly 33 million Migraineurs in the United States. This is more than the 32 million sufferers of asthma, diabetes, and coronary heart disease combined.*
  - *More than 7.5 million Migraineurs in the United Kingdom.*
  - *More than 4 million Migraineurs in Canada.*
- In developed countries, tension-type headache affects two-thirds of adult males and over 80 percent of females. Once again, let's see some numbers from those percentages:
  - *Nearly 200 million people in the United States.*
  - *More than 43 million people in the United Kingdom.*
  - *More than 23 million people in Canada.*
- Migraine attacks result in 112 million bedridden days per year for U.S. Migraineurs alone.
- The best estimate is that the cost to U.S. industry of absenteeism and reduced productivity due to Migraine is $13 billion per year.

■ It is also estimated that Migraineurs in the United States lose more than 157 million workdays each year.

■ Many people with Migraine disease also have clinical depression, which is also a disease. We don't fully understand the link between the two diseases, but this very strong statistic shows there clearly is a link: 47 percent of Migraineurs also have clinical depression. In the general population, that figure is only 17 percent.

The Most Common Types of Headaches and Migraine Disease

■ The most common type of head pain is **tension-type headache (TTH)**. The pain of a TTH is usually on both sides of the head. The pain has a pressing or tightening quality, often feeling like a band around the head. The pain is seldom made worse by physical activity, but it may be accompanied by tenderness of the head and/or muscles in the jaw, neck, scalp, and shoulders. It may also be accompanied by sensitivity to light or noise, but not both. In developed countries, TTH affects two-thirds of adult males and over 80 percent of females. In the United States alone, that's over 187 million people.

■ **Migraine** is a genetic neurological disease that produces flare-ups referred to as "Migraine attacks" or "Migraine episodes." Within the disease, there are different types of Migraine, subtypes of the disease:

• *Migraine without aura* is the most common type of Migraine. It usually consists of a moderate to severe headache that's made worse by physical activity. It's also accompanied by at least one of the following: nausea, vomiting, sensitivity to light, or sensitivity to sound.

- *Migraine with aura* differs from Migraine without aura in that it has an extra phase before the headache, the aura. The most commonly thought of Migraine aura is visual disturbances, but aura can also include hearing or smelling things that aren't actually present as well as other symptoms.
- *Abdominal Migraine* occurs mainly in children. It consists of abdominal pain, nausea, and vomiting.
- *Hemiplegic Migraine* can include a prolonged aura that can last for days or weeks, paralysis on one side of the body, impaired consciousness, plus the symptoms of Migraine with aura. Hemiplegic Migraine should not be treated with triptans. It can be frightening and difficult to diagnose because it has symptoms that can be thought to be stroke, epilepsy, or other conditions.
- *Basilar-type Migraine (BTM)* is Migraine with aura with a twist. The aura symptoms can be far different from those typical of Migraine with aura—and very frightening. The aura of BTM can include temporary blindness, impaired hearing, double vision, and numbness or prickly feelings. BTM should not be treated with triptans.
- *Retinal Migraine* is characterized by repeated attacks of visual disturbances in one eye only. Those disturbances can include "sparkling lights," small blank spots in the vision, or blindness. These symptoms are usually, but not always, followed by a headache and other symptoms of Migraine without aura. Before diagnosing retinal Migraine, it's essential that doctors rule out any other possible causes of visual problems.

▌ **Cluster headaches** are considered by many to be the most painful type of head pain. Cluster headaches are attacks of severe, one-sided pain around the eye or temple region. A single headache may last 15 to 180 minutes and occur from once every other day to eight or more times a day. Other symptoms that often occur on the same side as the pain are tearing, nasal congestion, eyelid swelling, runny nose, contraction of the pupil, and drooping of the eyelid.

■ **Rebound headaches, aka medication overuse headaches,** are a "darned-if-you-do, darned-if-you-don't" situation. They're actually caused by the very medications we take to relieve our headaches and Migraine attacks. If we take medication for the pain of a headache or Migraine or to abort a Migraine more than two or three days a week, our bodies can get used to the medication. Our bodies are smart, so they do what they did to get the medication in the first place—create a headache. If you pay close attention to your symptoms, it's not terribly difficult to distinguish between a rebound headache and a Migraine attack or cluster headache because the rebound headache is a headache without the other symptoms of a Migraine attack or cluster headache. However, it's more difficult to distinguish between a tension-type headache and a rebound headache. The only thing that stops rebound headaches is to stop taking the kinds of medications that started them in the first place.

There are other variations on the headaches and Migraines just discussed, but they're far less common. Those we've already discussed will give us a good foundation or an overview, if you will, for moving on to more detailed discussion. I hope the statistics were as eye-opening for you as they were to me when I first discovered them. For me, they helped dispel some of the feelings of aloneness and isolation. There really *were* people like me—*many* of them! Of course, none of us would wish our illness on anyone else, but it is comforting to know we are *not* alone.

A Summary of Migraine Disease and Headaches Through History

Headaches and Migraines have plagued people from the beginning of time. Seeking relief, people have gone to desperate measures. Among the most desperate is trepanation, the drilling of holes in the skull. Signs of trepanation have been found on Neolithic human skulls dating as early as 7000–3000 BC. It was once thought that early trepanations had been performed to release demons and evil spirits, but more recent research suggests that, even then, trepanation was performed for medical reasons.

One of the earliest written references to headache goes back to a Mesopotamian poem dated between 4000 and 3000 BC. What is often said to be the oldest medical manuscript, the Ebers Papyrus, discovered at Thebes, Egypt, and dating between 1534 and 3000 BC, describes several different types of headache and has twelve prescriptions for headache. Of one headache preparations, supposed to have been prepared by the revered mother-goddess Isis herself for the sun god Ra, the Ebers Papyrus says, "A sixth remedy that Isis made for Ra himself to eliminate the disease that is in his head: fruit of coriander . . . made into a mass, honey is mixed with it, the head is bandaged therewith so that it goes immediately well with him."

In ancient Egypt, a clay crocodile holding grain in its mouth was bound firmly to a patient's head with a strip of linen bearing the names of the gods. It's possible that some relief may have been produced with this technique because it may have compressed and cooled the scalp.

The Greek father of medicine, Hippocrates (470–410 BC), treated headache by bloodletting, leeches, or trepanation. He also recommended vomiting to expel headaches from the body. He described a shining light, usually in the right eye, followed by severe pain beginning in the temples and continuing to encompass the entire head and neck area.

Because of his descriptions, Aretaeus of Cappodocia (second century AD) is credited with "discovering" Migraine. The term *migraine* comes from the Greek word *hemicrania,* which was introduced by Galen, a Greek doctor (131–201 AD). He recommended treating headache by applying a live torpedo, an electric fish related to a skate or ray, to the forehead. He thought the electric current from the fish would "numb the senses" and take away the pain.

Then there was the ancient Arabian doctor Albucasis (936–1013 AD), who was a proponent of applying a hot iron to the afflicted head. If that didn't cure the headache, he then recommended cutting a hole above the temple and inserting a garlic clove into the hole for fifteen hours.

Skipping ahead a few centuries, Thomas Willis, considered to be the "father of neurology," was the first to theorize that "megrim" was caused by blood "estuating" (stagnating) in the vessels and distending them, thus producing head pain.

In 1886, Atlanta pharmacist John Pemberton's search for a quick headache cure provided what would be one of the most famous brand names ever to hit the modern advertising world, Coca-Cola. He took his concoction to Jacobs' Pharmacy and combined it with carbonated water. Customers who sampled it were so enthusiastic that the pharmacy was soon selling it at the soda fountain for five cents a glass, and Coke was born.

Now to the Present

Some of you reading this have probably thought about drilling or knocking a hole in your head to see if it would help relieve your pain. Some of you have probably literally knocked your heads against walls. We think and do desperate things when the pain is at its worst. But good news is here. Even though you may feel that you will never get a proper diagnosis or treatment, at least 95 percent of people with chronic headaches and Migraine disease can now be helped with effective preventive regimens. Has your doctor not told you this? Your doctor may not know. Unfortunately, many medical schools have been slow to catch up to the progress being made in the field, and medical school students spend very little time studying head pain disorders in the first place.

Stop and think, too, about all the different illnesses and diseases that your doctor treats. How on earth can one person be expected to stay up-to-date on all of them? Even if you've gone from your family doctor to a neurologist, a general practice neurologist is still in the position of having many, many illnesses, diseases, and injuries that he or she must know how to treat. Again, especially in today's medical practices, how can general practitioners stay up-to-date?

After more than thirty years of headaches and Migraine, I was so frustrated at the lack of successful treatment and the attitude of the doctors I'd seen that I decided to start researching the field myself. Before long, I had a list of important information that no doctor had ever told me. It was information that could have helped me make a difference in my own health *if someone had told me*. It was that realization that prompted me to start the "Headaches and Migraine" site at About.com (www.headaches.about.com). That's not to say that there aren't doctors who talk to their patients and try to educate them, but I'd seen neurologist after neurologist and hadn't been told much of anything.

When you finish this book, you'll have a basic understanding of some of the different types of head pain disorders, understand the importance of being an active participant on your own health care team, know when it's time to move on to a new doctor, feel less helpless, and have a new sense of just who should be in charge of your health care.

Dr. William B. Young of the Jefferson Headache Center in Philadelphia summed up educated patients and the role of educated patients in our health care very well. When asked about educated patients, he replied, "An educated patient is a better patient. I'd far rather have a treatment partner than a dishrag." Are you a dishrag? I used to be, but no more! When you finish this book, you won't be, either.

[*An educated patient is a better patient. I'd far rather have a treatment partner than a dishrag.*
—*Dr. William B. Young*]

When you finish this book, you'll also understand why there are six elements to proper headache and Migraine management:

1. Education.
2. Trigger identification and management: identifying what brings on your headaches or Migraine attacks and learning how to manage those triggers.
3. A good preventive regimen.
4. Appropriate abortives (medications that actually stop a Migraine attack rather than just masking the pain).
5. An emergency plan and pain management for times when abortives fail.
6. A strong support system.

Using This Book

I want you to be tough on this book. Get a pencil or pen, a highlighter, sticky notes, a notepad, whatever you need to make notes on your copy, to mark pages, and to jot down any notes or questions you may have. Don't hesitate to make margin notes or highlight passages. If any of the terms are unfamiliar to you, check the glossary in appendix A. This isn't meant to be a great work of literature. It's an informational tool to help you all. You can expect a few spots to be wisecracking and irreverent because that's part of how I cope with head pain. It's amazing how much help even a slightly warped sense of humor can be. (If I were writing for the Internet, at this point, I'd insert a smiley face.) If I'm doing my job well, parts of this book will make you smile, parts will make you angry, and parts will make you sad.

So, please find a comfy place to read and just relax with this book. Put it to work for you. Obviously, there's far more to headaches and Migraine disease than can fit here. In appendix B, you'll find a list of supplemental materials I've made available online. If you don't have Internet access, please check your local library. Most libraries now have computers with Internet access that area citizens can use.

Moving Forward

As I said earlier, I've had headaches and Migraines since I was six years old. Now, at the age of fifty, that means I've had them through childhood, adolescence, young adulthood, menopause, and into middle age. Now I agonize when my granddaughters have a Migraine. I tell you this so you'll know that I've been in situations similar to those many of you face, and I'm here to tell you life can be great even if you do have chronic headaches or Migraine disease. You *can* "Live Well." That, my friends, is my fondest wish for each of you. If you'd like to contact me, you may do so through my Web site, www.HelpForHeadaches.com.

L'Chaim! (To life!)
Teri

2

The Importance of Proper Diagnosis

Proper diagnosis isn't important only to you; it's important to your family, too. This story was shared with me by Suzanne Simons. After reading this, I find it especially appropriate that, after working in some other areas, she is now executive director of the National Headache Foundation.

SUZANNE'S STORY

As a child, I knew my mother had headaches, though they didn't have a specific name at the time. I just knew they were bad, and they kept her from doing things with the family. She spent countless hours in bed with a cold rag on her forehead, the window blinds shut, and instructions for my sister and me to be extra quite. Many times, my mother was unable to cook dinner or attend family celebrations. I have a distinct memory of one family vacation that my mother spent lying in the backseat of the car with a Migraine as she quietly urged my father, sister, and me to have a good time. As time went on, my mother went from doctor to doctor trying to find a name for this disease that was robbing her of her most productive years. One day, she was reading a health column in the newspaper and the topic was headaches, more specifically Migraines. Suddenly the symptoms she experienced, which were described in the paper, had a name: It was Migraine. That was the first step in my mother's journey to diagnosis and treatment. From that point, my mother found a physician who understood Migraine and was able to diagnose her disease and put her on a treatment plan that gave back her quality of life.

The importance of getting an accurate diagnosis cannot be overemphasized. Statistically, head pain is usually not an indication of an extremely serious or life-threatening condition, but why take chances? Head pain can be symptomatic of organic problems such as stroke, aneurysm, or tumor. It can also be symptomatic of illnesses including Lyme disease, meningitis, thyroid disease, encephalitis, polycystic kidney diseases, multiple sclerosis, and others. Someone has to be among the small percentage of people with those serious conditions, and if it's you or someone close to you, you want to find out sooner rather than later. In those cases, early diagnosis and treatment can make a very real difference in the prognosis.

Another reason to get an accurate diagnosis as soon as possible is so you can begin the right treatment immediately. Treatments for tension headaches, Migraine attacks, cluster headaches, posttraumatic headaches, and other head pain can vary significantly. Not having the right diagnosis can mean more time spent needlessly in pain or possibly taking medications that could be harmful if you've been diagnosed incorrectly. For example, if someone is diagnosed with Migraine disease but actually has hemiplegic or basilar-type Migraines, and that explicit subtype is not included in the diagnosis, Migraine-specific medications meant to actually stop the Migraine attack rather than just treating the pain (Imitrex, Maxalt, Zomig, Amerge, Axert, Frova, Relpax, DHE-45, Migranal) could be prescribed. This could create a problem because such medications should not be prescribed for Migraineurs with hemiplegic or basilar-type Migraines. Those medications work in part by constricting blood vessels (making them smaller), and that puts Migraineurs with hemiplegic or basilar-type Migraine at higher risk for stroke.

A patient's participation is absolutely critical to an accurate diagnosis. There are no diagnostic tests that allow doctors to simply and accurately diagnose tension headaches, cluster headaches, Migraine disease, or other head pain disorders. They're diagnosed by reviewing medical history, family medical history, and symptoms and conducting a thorough physical examination. When tests are ordered, they're ordered to rule out other conditions. Thus, a great deal of the information our doctors need to provide an accurate diagnosis must come directly from you. Since family medical history can play a role in the diagnosis of head pain, a bit of homework is in order. It's so easy to think you're prepared but draw a blank or realize you've missed things once you're at the doctor's office filling out that history paperwork. To get you started, I've set up a medical history checklist you'll find at the end of this chapter (or that can be printed from www.HelpForHeadaches.com/lwfiles/history-checklist. htm). As you think about it, use the back of it to note anything else that you think could possibly be relevant. The form asks about the history of your blood relatives and your personal medical history as well as about any tests you may already have had. If you've had a CAT (computerized tomography) scan, MRI, or other imaging studies fairly recently, you can get copies of them to take with you to the doctor, possibly saving yourself the time and expense of new ones. If you don't know the medical history of your birth family, you obviously can't do much about that part of the medical history. Don't stress about it. If there's a way to get the information, do so. If not, just let it go and work on your personal medical history.

Another great tool, both for diagnosis and for working on a treatment regimen, is a head pain diary that records the date and time that you experience head pain, the pain level, the impact of the pain on your daily activity, and other information. (See sample on page 19.) This diary can be an invaluable tool to your doctor from your first visit on through your treatment. Obviously the sample here in the book isn't large enough to use, but I've put the diary on-line for you in three formats: printable to fill in by hand, Microsoft Word format to use on your computer, and Microsoft Excel format with sample graphing to use on your computer. You can find the dairies at www.HelpForHeadaches.com/lwfiles/diaries.htm.

The place most people start in getting a diagnosis is with their primary care physician (PCP). Quite often, the PCP will refer headache and Migraine patients to a neurologist because the PCP treats so many different conditions that he or she feels a specialist is better qualified to handle some cases. This is very common and shouldn't be alarming to you. If your PCP struggles with your diagnosis, don't hesitate to ask to be referred to a neurologist.

Unfortunately, we don't always get the appropriate and correct diagnosis the first time around. Answers not to accept:

- "It's all stress. Learn to relax."
- "Get pregnant. Your headaches will stop."
- "Have a hysterectomy. Your Migraines will go away."
- "Congratulations. You're an intellectual and have Migraines. Take some acetaminophen." (Seriously, a doctor told me that once!)
- "Just wait for menopause. Then they'll stop."
- "You're too high-strung and have a headache personality. See a psychiatrist."
- "It's a woman thing."
- "If triptans don't work, it's not a Migraine."

- ▌ "It's just something you'll have to learn to live with."
- ▌ "Just take a nap when you get a headache."
- ▌ "Stop taking everything so seriously."

Should you encounter any of these answers, your first reaction may be to strike the person making the statement. Please restrain yourself. You'll only cause yourself more problems in the long run. No, take the high road. Politely tell the doctor that his or her services will no longer be needed, then leave. If you've been a patient of that doctor for a long enough period of time to want a copy of your records, on your way out ask one of the office staff about getting a copy. If you're in the United States, provisions in HIPAA (Health Insurance Portability and Accountability Act) state that they must provide you with a copy within thirty days. They may charge you a "reasonable" fee for copies, but they must give you the copy, and they cannot insist upon sending it to another doctor instead. Remember, this is your head, your pain, your health. The doctor isn't paying you; you're paying the doctor. You are entitled to the same respect that the doctor expects. There's always another doctor out there for a second opinion. We'll discuss finding the right doctor in more depth in chapter 10.

Headache and Migraine Diary

Impact on activity ratings: 1–10 (less > more)
Intensity of pain ratings: 1–10 (lowest > highest)

Date Time HA/Migraine	Impact	Intensity	Medication Taken	Dosage	Time to Relief	Triggers	Comments

Headache and Migraine Diary

Impact on activity ratings: 1–10 (less > more)
Intensity of pain ratings: 1–10 (lowest > highest)

Date Time HA/Migraine	Impact	Intensity	Medication Taken	Dosage	Time to Relief	Triggers	Comments

Health History Checklist

You can also find this online at www.HelpForHeadaches.com/lwfiles/
history-checklist.htm.

Do you know of a blood relative who has had:
___ Arthritis
___ Alcohol/substance abuse problems
___ Asthma
___ Cancer
___ Depression
___ Diabetes
___ Epilepsy/seizure disorder
___ Headache (tension-type, cluster, other)
___ Heart disease
___ Hypertension
___ Kidney/renal disease
___ Liver disease
___ Migraine disease
___ Psychiatric disease
___ Sinus headaches
___ Stroke/transient ischemic attack
___ Thyroid disease

Have you ever had any of the following:
___ Arthritis
___ Alcohol/substance abuse problems
___ Asthma
___ Cancer
___ Cervical neck/spine problems
___ Deep vein thrombosis/phlebitis
___ Dental problems
___ Depression

___ Diabetes

___ Ear, nose, and throat problems

___ Epilepsy/seizure disorder

___ Glaucoma

___ Gynecological problems

___ Head injury

___ Headache (tension-type, cluster, other)

___ Heart disease

___ Hypertension

___ Insomnia/problems with sleep

___ Infectious diseases

___ Kidney/renal disease

___ Psychiatric disease

___ Pulmonary disease

___ Sinus headaches

___ Skin problems

___ Stroke/transient ischemic attack

___ Thyroid disease

___ Ulcers/gastrointestinal problems

___ Other _____

___ Other _____

3

Education: Essential to Our Health and Well-Being

> *The best prescription is knowledge.*
> *—Former Surgeon General*
> *Dr. C. Everett Koop*

If struck by some illnesses and diseases, we're pretty much at the mercy of the illness or disease and doctors. There's not much we can do to control the disease or the level of control it gains over our lives. That's an unfortunate and sometimes tragic fact of life. On the other hand, with Migraine disease and other head pain disorders, there are often many things we can do to control them instead of allowing them to control our lives. That's a positive!

Our best tool and ally in gaining and retaining as much control as possible is—drumroll, please—*knowledge*. That makes *education* number one on our list of the six elements to proper headache and Migraine management. Someone I said that to once thought I meant we all had to go back to school and take some medical classes. No way! There are no classes that would offer the information we need. That's a shame, but that's also different topic. As we take a look at education in this chapter, you may want to know more. Never fear! This chapter is like an introduction to the educational issues we need to address. Everything I mention here is covered in more depth in later chapters.

What Do We Need to Learn?

I could tell you we need to learn everything possible, but that wouldn't be very helpful, would it? So I'll list some areas in which we need to educate ourselves. We're all different, so each of us may need to learn more in some areas than others, and we may find an area that I don't even list. We can at least start with these areas:

- *The types of headaches and/or Migraines we experience.* We discussed this earlier when we talked about the importance of a proper diagnosis. In chapters 4 through 8, we'll discuss various types of headaches and different forms of Migraine disease. Many people experience more than one. For example, it's not unusual for a person to have both tension-type headaches and Migraine with or without aura. Learning all we can about any form of head pain that affects us helps us gain power and control over it.
- *How to be an effective member of our health care team.* We're the ones walking around with heads that often feel as if they're going to explode. Our health care team will be incomplete and not as effective as possible unless we're an effective member of that team. We'll discuss that in detail in chapter 9.
- *Doctors.* What is reasonable to expect from a doctor? How do we choose a doctor? These are also things about which we need to educate ourselves. Again, we'll go into more detail on this (see chapter 10).

■ *Trigger identification and management.* Do you know how to identify triggers? How about managing them once you identify them? Of course, there are some that can't really be managed very well, but just knowing what our triggers are can be an enormous help. Learning how to identify and manage triggers can make an enormous difference in our lives.

■ *Medications.* This is an area where the learning is never-ending. Think you've tried all the medications available? Think again. Just today, someone told me about a medication that was helping her with Migraine prevention. I'd never heard of it being used for Migraine prevention before. There are actually two areas of learning here:

- **The medications prescribed for us.** Whenever a new medication is prescribed for us, we need to learn all we can about it.

- **Medication options.** There's no way doctors can keep up with everything. Headache and Migraine specialists will be better versed on the medication options available to us because headache and Migraine are all they treat. Family doctors and general practice neurologists don't stand a chance because they have so many illnesses and diseases to treat. Even when a doctor knows a certain medication is being used for headache and Migraine, he or she may not know the dosing being used. If we're educating ourselves, we'll probably have information from a reliable source that we can share with them.

■ *Terminology.* "In plain English, please?!" How many times have we said or thought that? If you're reading this book, the chances are pretty good that your headaches or Migraine disease are not short-term. Learning a bit of the medical terminology we're likely to hear frequently can be exceedingly helpful. What do unilateral, photophobia, and hemiplegia mean? In addition to medical terms, there are medical abbreviations and abbreviations used in writing prescriptions. If you don't understand a word used in this book, please check appendix A, the glossary. Overall, there are some great medical dictionaries as well as books to help understand pharmacology terms and others.

▎ *We all need support.* We need to learn about the various support options available to us, how to access them, and which ones are most comfortable for us. We also need to learn how to build and maintain a solid support system for ourselves.

▎ *Our rights.* There are times when we need to know our rights as patients or as employees. Did you know our doctors are required to provide us with a copy of our medical records if we request them? Do you know how the Family and Medical Leave Act (FMLA) works? There may come a time when any one of us needs to educate herself on these issues.

How Do We Educate Ourselves?

▎ *Listen to our doctors and ask questions.* Some doctors will be willing to loan us relevant medical journals to read. If we don't have doctors with whom this will work, it's time to change doctors. You'll find more about that in chapter 10.

▎ *Talk to our pharmacist* about the medications prescribed for us.

▎ *Read and save prescription information sheets.* When we fill prescriptions, our pharmacist should include a patient information sheet with the medication. It's a good idea to not only read, but save, these sheets for reference purposes.

It's easy to forget what they said, especially if we're taking multiple medications.

▮ *Check to see if there's a local support group.* Local support groups sometimes have speakers who are excellent educational resources. You can find more about this in chapter 18.

▮ *Be alert for television programming.* There have been some decent stories on network television lately. They don't have all their facts straight, but they're getting better. The Discovery Health Channel has a couple of very good and informative headache and Migraine programs they run periodically that feature excellent specialists. As I write this, another major cable network has a series of programs on headache and Migraine in the works. They're collaborating with an excellent headache and Migraine specialist, so I know the series will be accurate and valuable.

▮ *Check out magazine articles.* They're not always totally accurate, but they seem to be getting better. Take what's there with a grain of salt, and read them discriminatingly. Remember what you've learned previously. Jot down any questions they raise so you can get them answered.

▮ *Read some books.* Where you can find books will depend greatly upon where you live. Some libraries will have current books, some won't. If you live near a university, check to see if they offer public access to their library. Some offer access for reading in the library only. Others allow local citizens to check out books as well. Bookstores are fine, but obviously they can't carry every book available. If you don't find what you want, ask a salesperson to review books that are available by special order. Online book stores have the advantages of more available titles, reviews by other readers, and often lower prices.

Note: If a book promises a "cure" for Migraine disease or says Migraine is psychological in origin, make a note of the author and don't waste your time reading anything by that person. At this time, there is *no* cure for Migraine disease, and Migraines are neurological, *not* psychological.

You'll find a variety of books. Some will be written by doctors, some by fellow sufferers. Each will have its strengths. One thing to check is the copyright date. There has been so much progress in the field of headache and Migraine that if books are very old, they may well contain outdated information. I don't want to appear to be critical of anyone's work, so I'll just say there's a popular book by an excellent person in the field that people are still buying even though the copyright date is 1990, before the introduction of triptans in the United States and well before current imaging technology allowed doctors to observe the brain during a Migraine attack and develop the most current theories about the true cause of Migraine. Thus, although parts of that book are still relevant, parts of it are woefully out-of-date. You'll also find there are books written for patients and books written for doctors. Once you've educated yourself a bit, some of the books written for doctors will not be above your level of comprehension. You may need to have a medical dictionary available and occasionally research something you find in these books, but some are quite readable for an educated patient. Some of these books are listed in appendix D ("Recommended Reading"). They are more expensive, but you can often buy used copies through various sources, including Amazon.com.

■ *Surf the Web* for good and accurate Internet sites. Notice I said "good and accurate." Unfortunately, there are too many inaccurate sites and sites that are there just to try to sell a dubious product or get you to enter into a multilevel marketing program. If something seems too good to be true, it most likely is. Here are some things to look for in a "good" Web site:

- Is it fairly easy to tell who wrote the content and how to contact them?
- Is the information given backed by both scientific and anecdotal data? If too much is backed only by anecdotal data, be wary.
- When scientific/study data is referred to, is it cited properly?
- If there are claims of a "cure," forget it.
- If it's a Migraine site, does the content make it clear that Migraine is a disease?
- If the site refers to "headache personality" or "Migraine personality" or suggests that headaches or Migraines are psychological in origin, don't waste your time.
- Is the site kept up-to-date, with new content added on a regular basis? There's new information coming to light in this field quite often. If a Web site sits unchanged for long periods of time, it can't be considered to be dependable information.
- If the site is one that asks visitors to register, is there a privacy policy clearly stated?
- If the site makes claims that seem too good to be true, they probably are.
- Appendix C of this book offers a list of recommended Web sites you can trust. These are good sites to begin with.

▐ *Watch for seminars, lectures, classes, and workshops.* Increasingly, there are such events occurring for patients and other people who are interested. Some are conducted by one person, some by a panel. There is often a question and answer period at the end that can prove very helpful.

As you can see, there are many opportunities and methods for educating ourselves. We just need to watch for and take advantage of them. Education *will* help us along the path toward controlling our headaches and Migraines.

4

The Most Common Headache: Tension Headaches

EXAMPLE CASE *Aaron's head pain sometimes starts in the back of his head, near the base of his skull. Sometimes it begins in his forehead. He describes it as vise-like or as if someone has taken his tie, tied it around his head, and is pulling it very tight. He does not experience nausea, vomiting, or sensitivity to light or sound. Physical activity does not aggravate the pain. When he's at home, a hot shower and a caffeinated beverage will sometimes relieve his headache. When that doesn't work or isn't an option, ibuprofen and caffeine are his first choices for treatment. Should those fail, he does have prescription pain medication to use.*

According to the World Health Organization (WHO), in developed countries tension-type headaches affect two-thirds of adult males and over 80 percent of females. In the United States alone, that's nearly 200 million people. That makes tension headaches the most common type of headache. Chronic tension-type headaches (tension headaches more than 180 days per year) affect approximately 4.5 percent of our population. Dr. William Young of the Jefferson Headache Center in Philadelphia states, "At least 80 percent of us will have a tension headache at some time in our lives."

Symptoms of Tension-Type Headache

▌ The pain is usually on both sides of the head, but it may be anywhere on the head.

▌ The pain is of a pressing/tightening quality, often described as band-like, dull, pressing, or aching.

▌ The pain is unilateral (one-sided) in approximately 20 percent of patients.

▌ The pain is usually mild to moderate (enough pain to inhibit but not prohibit activities).

▌ The pain can last from thirty minutes to seven days.

▌ Tenderness of the head.

▌ Tenderness of the muscles of the jaw, neck, scalp, and shoulders.

▌ Difficulty concentrating.

▌ Heightened sensitivity to light or noise, but not both.

Symptoms *missing* in TTH:

▌ Typical physical activity seldom intensifies pain.

▌ Migraine prodrome symptoms such as food cravings, increased appetite, mood changes, muscle stiffness, fatigue, yawning. The prodrome is the first of four possible phases of a Migraine attack. We'll look at it more closely in chapter 5.

▌ Migraine aura symptoms such as visual disturbances, smelling or hearing things that aren't actually present, tingling of the hands or lips, inability to speak correctly. The aura is the second of four possible phases of a Migraine attack. We'll look at it more closely in chapter 5.

▌ Nausea and vomiting.

▌ Diarrhea.

▌ Heightened sensitivity to light and noise (one may be present).

Here's a key fact that you'll see throughout this book:

> One size does not fit all. Within a given head pain disorder, there will be variations and subtypes, as well as variations from one person to the next.

As with other headache disorders, there are no definitive diagnostic tests that can be used to say, "Aha! This person has tension-type headaches!" Diagnosis is made based on medical history; symptoms; neurological examination; and ruling out organic disorders such as aneurysm, stroke, or brain tumor. If you've kept a diary with notes of your symptoms and other information, that will be helpful to your doctor in arriving at a diagnosis.

For most people, TTH occurs only periodically, and relief can be achieved with an over-the-counter pain reliever, an ice pack, and perhaps a nap. Massage, meditation, and relaxation exercises are also helpful for some people. When they occur more frequently, however, they acquire slightly different names:

▌ Infrequent episodic tension-type headache: TTH occurring less than 12 days per year.

▌ Frequent episodic tension-type headache: at least ten episodes occurring on more than 1 but fewer than 15 days per month for at least 3 months (more than 12 and fewer than 180 days per year).

▌ Chronic tension-type headache: headache occurring on 15

or more days per month on average for more than 3 months (180 or more days per year). Chronic tension-type headache evolves over time from episodic tension-type headache.

The difference in name/diagnosis is especially helpful if you change doctors or are treated away from home. These diagnostic classifications come from the International Headache Society (IHS) "International Classification of Headache Disorders," a system universally accepted in the field to help standardize diagnosis and classification rather than every doctor or group of doctors calling different types of head pain disorders by different names.

It's theorized that sufferers of TTH have a genetic predisposition to their headaches, but the actual cause of TTH is really unknown. Older theories suggested that muscle tension caused them. At one point, tension-type headaches were actually called muscle contraction headaches. More recent research indicates that during a TTH, there is actually more muscle tenderness than muscle tension. The most current theory of the root cause of TTH is stated in Silberstein et al.'s *Headache in Primary Care:* "TTH is now believed to result from abnormal neuronal sensitivity and pain facilitation, not abnormal muscle contraction."

The onset of TTH is often late afternoon, when the day's stress has reached its peak. In addition to stress, other triggers can include sleep deprivation, eyestrain, and bad posture. When the onset is early in the day, not enough sleep or poor-quality sleep is often suspected, and a sleep study may be helpful. For a sleep study, the night is spent at a sleep laboratory, which is often part of a hospital but set apart a bit so it's quieter than the average hospital floor. In some labs, in an effort to more closely simulate the patient's home sleeping conditions, the rooms are more like those in a hotel than a hospital. Electrodes are attached to the scalp and limbs to record brain activity and limb movement. A camera in the room tapes the patient during the night. All of this enables the doctor evaluating the study to determine how much sleep the patient gets during the night, how much time is spent in each stage of sleep, the overall quality of sleep, and if there are any sleep disorders that should be addressed.

Overall, tension-type headaches are the most common and the most harmless type of headache. However, that doesn't mean we should self-diagnose or not seek treatment. Even if you think it's "just a headache," there are times you need to mention it to your doctor:

▪ If you're experiencing headaches twice a month or more on a regular basis.

▪ If a dose of an over-the-counter analgesic and some rest don't relieve your headache.

▪ If you have other symptoms such as nausea, vomiting, sensitivity to light and sound, any visual disturbances, or muscle weakness along with the head pain.

▪ If your headaches increase in frequency or severity.

▪ Anytime you have a severe headache, that's the "worst headache of your life."

Please let these two examples serve to show the importance of seeking medical care:

▪ When actress Sharon Stone appeared on *The Oprah Winfrey Show* in July 2004, she shared a frightening experience with the audience. She has Migraines, but the pain she felt one night was different. She said she just didn't feel right, so she called her ex-husband to ask him to take her to the emergency room. He wasn't in, so she left him a message. By that time, she was disoriented and not thinking clearly. It turns out that her ex was out of town, and she spent the next three days wandering around her house before he came to check on her. When she arrived at the hospital, they learned that she had an aneurysm that had been bleeding into her head all that time. She nearly died. We need to heed her warning: "If you have the worst headache you've ever had, go to the hospital, because by the time you get to the hospital, you're as far gone as you wanna be."

▌ Singer Laura Branigan died in her sleep in August, 2004. She had no prior history of headaches or Migraine disease. Her brother told reporters that she had been complaining of a headache for about two weeks but had not sought medical care. The cause of death? A cerebral aneurysm. Had she sought care when she first started experiencing the headache, there's a good chance she'd be alive today.

Don't let yourself or anyone else make you feel silly for going to the doctor for a headache. It may be "just a headache," but you don't know until you get it checked out. The risks are too big to avoid seeking a diagnosis. I know of some doctors who dismissed headaches when the patient had a true headache disorder that needed treatment. Hopefully your doctor wouldn't do that, but if that ever happens to you, don't hesitate to get a second opinion. A good doctor will respect your wishes for a second opinion and not be offended. Remember, we are ultimately the ones responsible for our own health and our own health care.

5

Migraine Disease: Migraines Are Not "Just Bad Headaches"

According to the World Health Organization, 6 percent of men and 18 percent of women have Migraine disease. When those prevalence statistics are applied to the last official U.S. census, they add up to nearly 33 million American Migraineurs.

Many people continue to think Migraines are "just bad headaches." If they have headaches, they tend to call their mild headaches "headaches" and their more severe headaches "Migraines." That's just plain incorrect. In fact, Migraines aren't headaches, strictly speaking. We now know that Migraine is a genetic neurological disease that flares up when we encounter triggers and produces Migraine attacks. Sometimes one of the *symptoms* of a Migraine attack is a headache, but it is only one of the *symptoms*, not the attack itself, and not all Migraine attacks include a headache.

Researchers are working to identify the genes responsible for this disease. At this point, the genes for familial hemiplegic Migraine have been identified, and research continues to identify the genes responsible for other forms of Migraine disease.

Saying that it's genetic or inherited can be confusing because some people may not remember anyone in their family having a history of Migraine. However, with a bit of detective work, Migraineurs will almost always find someone in their family history who suffered "sick headaches" or severe "sinus headaches." Research over the last couple of years indicates that as much as 90 percent of self-diagnosed sinus headaches are actually Migraine attacks. Unless there's an infection present, it's actually unusual for the sinuses to present a headache.

Migraine is a genetic neurological disease. It's as much a disease as diabetes, epilepsy, or thyroid disease; and it's time it started being treated as such.

There are still multiple theories of what actually occurs to cause a Migraine attack when we encounter a trigger. But advancements in imaging technology have allowed scientists to observe the brain during a Migraine episode. The most prevalent theory is that Migraineurs have overly excitable neurons (nerve cells that have the ability to transmit and receive nervous impulses) in our brains. When we encounter a trigger, those neurons fire in a wave across the brain, starting a cascade of events involving several centers of the brain, including the brain stem. The end of that cascade involves dilation or swelling of the blood vessels in the brain and the surrounding tissues, accompanied by inflammation of small arteries in the coverings of the brain. The headache of a Migraine attack, if there is one, is from sensory impulses transmitted by the nerves from these inflamed blood vessels and surrounding tissues transmitted to higher centers of the brain and experienced as pain. Others believe the initial event occurs in what has been called the Migraine generator in the brain stem, which initiates the attack and causes changes in levels of chemical messengers (neurotransmitters), including serotonin.

The Phases of a Migraine Attack

A Migraine attack can consist of up to four distinct phases. Once again, one size does not fit all. Not all Migraineurs experience all the phases, and one Migraine can vary from the next.

▌ *Prodrome* phase: The prodrome is a kind of premonitory phase that can occur from an hour to two days before any headache occurs. Prodrome symptoms are more annoying than anything else, but the 30–40 percent of Migraineurs who experience this phase can learn to be more aware of the symptoms and use the prodrome phase to their advantage by seeing it as advance warning of what is to come in a Migraine attack. Prodrome symptoms may include:
  - *food cravings*
  - *increased appetite*
  - *constipation or diarrhea*
  - *mood changes—depression, irritability, euphoria, and the like*
  - *muscle stiffness, especially in the neck*
  - *fatigue, drowsiness*
  - *increased frequency of urination*
  - *yawning*
  - *difficulty concentrating*
  - *stiff neck*
  - *aphasia (loss or impairment of the power to use or comprehend words)*
  - *dysphasia (impairment of speech)*
▌ *Aura* phase: Approximately 20 percent of Migraineurs experience the aura phase of a Migraine. The aura is probably one of the most misunderstood parts of Migraine. Those who don't experience Migraines seem to think the aura

phase is something we all experience. Even some doctors have told patients that they can't be having Migraines because they don't have the aura. For those who experience aura, it generally occurs with some Migraine attacks; in fewer cases, it occurs with every Migraine attack. The aura is a complex of widely varying reversible neurological symptoms that develop over a period of five to sixty minutes. Reversible means that the symptoms end with the end of the aura or Migraine. If they persist beyond that, you should consult your doctor. There are several different types of aura:

- *Visual aura is the most common form. It can manifest itself in various ways: scintillation, which is the perception of twinkling light of varying intensity; scotoma, which is the occurrence of an area or areas of decreased or lost vision, sometimes called "Swiss cheese" vision; wavy or zig-zag lines; and other variations.*

- *The second most common type of aura is a sensory aura consisting of a tingling feeling or numbness, generally beginning in a hand or near the lips. Please note that there is a difference between tingling/numbness and paralysis. Paralysis during a Migraine is totally different and needs to be brought to your doctor's attention immediately.*

- *Olfactory hallucinations: Some Migraineurs will smell odors that aren't actually present. Some are pleasant, some aren't.*

- *Auditory hallucinations: Some Migraineurs will hear sounds that aren't actually present. It can be music playing, a clock ticking, the sound of footsteps, just about anything.*

- *Aphasia, the inability to speak correctly, especially to remember the correct words for what one wants to say, can also be part of a Migraine aura.*

- *"Alice in Wonderland" syndrome: This rare form of aura occurs more frequently in children than adults and consists of visual alterations and distortions in body image and perspective. This aura was given its name from the imagery in Lewis Carroll's* Alice's Adventures in Wonderland *and* Through the Looking-Glass, and What Alice Found There. *It's known that Carroll was a Migraineur, and it is thought that much of the imagery in his books may have come from his own Migraine auras.*

■ *Headache* phase: The headache phase usually lasts from four to seventy-two hours and can consist of a headache as well as other symptoms. Some people experience Migraine attacks without the headache. Such Migraines are referred to by several terms, including acephalgic Migraine, silent Migraine, and Migraine variant. The symptoms of the headache phase can include

- *headache:*
  - The pain is usually, though not always, unilateral—on one side.
  - The pain level is generally moderate to severe.
  - Rather than a steady ache, the pain is usually, though not always, pulsatile—throbbing and pulsing.
  - Physical activity aggravates the pain.
- *nausea and/or vomiting, diarrhea*
- *dizziness*
- *allodynia—sensitivity to touch that would otherwise be pleasant or nonpainful*
- *phonophobia—increased sensitivity to sound*
- *photophobia—increased sensitivity to light*
- *loss of appetite or food cravings*
- *rhinorrhea—runny nose*
- *lacrimation—tearing of one or both eyes*

- *nasal congestion*
- *hot flashes and chills*
- *dehydration or fluid retention*
- *inability to concentrate*
- *confusion*
- *an array of emotions that can be totally irrational: fear, depression, anxiety, nervousness, irritability, even total panic*

▌ *Postdrome* phase (sometimes called postheadache): Once the headache is over, the Migraine episode is still not over. The postdrome follows immediately afterward. The majority of Migraineurs take hours to fully recover; some take days. Many people describe postdrome as feeling "like a zombie" or "hung-over." These feelings are often attributed to medications taken to treat the Migraine but may well be caused by the Migraine itself. Postdromal symptoms have been shown to be accompanied and possibly caused by abnormal cerebral blood flow and EEG (electroencephalogram) readings for up to twenty-four hours after the end of the headache stage. In cases where prodrome and/or aura are experienced without the headache phase, the postdrome may still occur. Symptoms of postdrome can include

- *lowered mood levels, especially depression, or feelings of well-being and euphoria*
- *fatigue*
- *poor concentration and comprehension*
- *scalp tenderness*

Migraine Disease and Children

One of the most hateful, insidious things about Migraine disease is that it can and does strike children, even some who are too young to be able to tell us what's wrong. It was bad enough that I had my first Migraine attack at the age of six, but one of our granddaughters wasn't even three-years-old when she suffered her first attack.

Below is an interview excerpt from www.migraines.org with Michael John Coleman, founder and executive director of MAGNUM, the National Migraine Association, in which he discusses his childhood experiences with Migraine disease. If you are a young person reading this book, his childhood experiences may sound familiar to you. He and I both hope you feel better knowing that you are not alone. However, if you are not getting medical care now, please make sure you sit down with your parents and ask for help. You don't have to try to "just live with" this horrible disease. Understanding your illness as well as working with your parents and a good doctor will get you on the road to enjoying more of your life! If you're a parent with a child Migraineur, this may give you better insight into what your child experiences. Michael John is also an award-winning artist, and his artistry comes through in his narrative, making it vivid and real.

Dancing with Migraine Disease as a Youth
By Michael John Coleman

I still remember clearly the first time a Migraine disrupted my life. I was just six-years-old and in the first grade. I looked sick enough that the teacher asked me to put my head down on my desk. I still recall looking through the tall classroom windows, with the blinds drawn all the way up and dark battleship-gray fluffy-bellied clouds looming as part of an approaching autumn thunderstorm. Unbeknownst to me at the time was that atmospheric pressure changes, induced by weather fronts, was a major Migraine trigger, a fact I would learn later in life. I marveled as the clouds seemed to hover

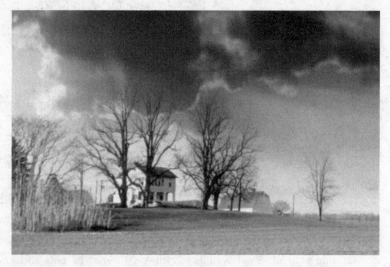

USDA Roadside View © Michael John Coleman 1978

over one side of the playground and the bright and painful af-
ternoon sunlight on the opposite side of a baseball field, a
chiaroscuro effect.

To this day, dramatic skies play a dominant role in the
landscapes I produce as an artist. The pain of my Migraines
throughout my life has been like being tortured by invisible
terrorists. An acute, severe Migraine is difficult to explain to a
nonsufferer. Put it this way: After enduring the so-called
headaches, you don't fear other things such as dentists and
bullies. But you do fear having to explain to your childhood
friends why you don't want to go out to play basketball. Bet-
ter to play in pain than say, "I have a headache," as that just
invites bullying because kids just don't understand what they
have not experienced.

Growing up didn't make things any easier; my Migraines
just became more aggressive as I entered puberty. However, I
learned tricks to cope socially. In a Washington, D.C., subur-

ban high school, I had some great friends; only a few knew I had sick headaches (as they were often called "back in the day"). The pain was horrible, the flickering fluorescent lights in the classrooms made me feel as if I were being hit on the head with each flutter. No one else understood, so many teachers opened the blinds on sunny days, and within fifteen minutes the glaring sunlight would beckon the Migraine's aura as it would come dancing into my line of sight. Never painful, the aura, but it was like Alice's Cheshire Cat, as it loved taunting me, letting me know I was not going to make it through the class.

The nausea would come next. That sick feeling in my gut wanted to make me vomit, but not in front of my classmates. The pounding would start, like being hit by a baseball bat every thirty or forty seconds. It was amazing that I passed my classes! The pain would get so bad that I would grab a clump of my hair and pull as hard as I could to distract myself from the pain. I felt like I was going to rip a patch of scalp from my head, but luckily for me I still have all my hair. I would suffer wave after wave of nausea, and I felt like if I could just vomit, I would feel so much better. But never in the classroom in front of the healthy kids, no never that.

Never that, because sick people are weak in the eyes of a high school child, and weakness makes you a target of abuse. Luckily for me, it was the 1970s and illegal drugs were cool, so I would make a beeline to the boys' room when the bell rang. I looked like I had been up all night, in a cold sweat, and would kick the door open and head right for a toilet. Often the pain was so bad I would be shaking, and in the spirit of Regan in The Exorcist I would spew projectile vomit across the bathroom floor. Not a pretty sight. Others would walk in behind me, and as I sat on the floor throwing up into a toilet, I could often hear my peers comment, "Hey, Cole-

man's so wasted, he's cool, man!" Like I said, luckily for me, it was the 1970s, so I was "in," and never did I let them know I was really severely ill. After severe vomiting, I'd feel a bit better, at least for a short while, until about halfway through my next class when the fun would begin again.

I had many friends back then who never had experienced head pain of any type, and I still know many people like that today, who never understand suffering. Or oddly enough, who never even figure out I am in violent pain so often. It's amazing to me as an adult today to know so many good and decent people who don't have a clue what a person in pain deals with.

As an adult, the pain and suffering I have lived through is frightening, and what is more frightening is knowing that there are millions of others who face this and lose millions of days, weeks, and even years of their lives to Migraine disease. It is only through good disease education, good treatment, proper treatment, and fighting to reclaim my life that I feel alive today. It amazes me that I still marvel at those dramatic summer thunderclouds with all their beauty, knowing that the barometric pressure change they bring with them may make me horribly ill. But at least now there are things I can do to fight back.

Mr. Coleman's words paint quite a picture for us. Since he and I first experienced Migraines at the same age, his story brings back many memories of childhood Migraine attacks for me as well as reminding me of my adult struggles. We'll discuss Migraine treatment for children in later chapters.

At this point, you may be thinking Migraine disease is more complex than you realized. If so, you're not alone. It's far more complex than I originally realized, and I learn new bits of information all the time.

This is a good place to point out the inaccuracy of the phrase "Migraine headache," as it's commonly used. The phrase is usually used instead of "Migraine attack." Since you've just read about the phases of a Migraine attack, you now know that the headache, if one even occurs, is but one symptom, not the actual Migraine attack. This may seem like a small matter, but if we stop referring to Migraines as "headaches" or "Migraine headaches," it will help educate people to the fact that Migraine is a genetic neurological disease and a Migraine attack consists of far more than a headache.

One of the many things that can be confusing about Migraine is the areas in which Migraineurs experience pain. Why do the sinuses hurt? The eyes? The ears? The jaw? The trigeminal nerve is affected by Migraine attacks, and it has three branches that go to various parts of the facial area. You can see an illustration of this at www.HelpForHeadaches.com/lwfiles/pathways.htm.

Types of Migraine

Within the disease, there are different types of Migraine. Some are minor variations, but others have characteristics that make them a more serious matter and make a big difference in the medications that can be prescribed for the Migraineurs who experience them. The different types of Migraine include the following:

Migraine without Aura

EXAMPLE CASE #1: *Brenda sometimes suspects a Migraine attack is coming before she experiences any pain because she yawns a lot and has problems finding the right words for what she wants to say in conversations (aphasia). Sometimes family and close friends will notice her prodrome before she does because they notice the aphasia in their conversations. In most of her Migraine attacks, nausea and pain strike at approximately the same time, along with extreme photophobia (sensitivity to light) and moderate phonophobia (sensitivity to sound). Her head pain has always been unilateral, at her temple with some supraorbital (just above the orbit of the eye) pain. The pain is pulsatile (seems to throb with her pulse). Triptans work well for her, and when taken early in a Migraine attack, one dose will usually abort a Migraine completely. If she doesn't medicate early in the attack, it often takes two doses and sleep to give her relief.*

EXAMPLE CASE #2: *Craig has so far not been able to identify any prodrome symptoms. His first indication of a Migraine attack is usually sudden and severe nausea, followed very shortly by unilateral, pulsatile head pain. His symptoms often include ipsilateral (on the same side as the headache) sinus pain, vertigo, photophobia, and tearing. Craig has severe, uncontrolled hypertension (high blood pressure), so triptans are not a treatment option for him. At the onset of his nausea, he immediately takes an antinausea drug such as Phenergan. For relief of the pain, he uses a compound analgesic such as acetaminophen with hydrocodone. Unfortunately, he still often vomits and must use antiemetic suppositories to stop the vomiting. After a Migraine, he describes himself as feeling "hung-over," which indicates postdrome symptoms.*

Previously called "common Migraine," this is the most common type of Migraine. Migraine without aura would, of course, skip the aura phase described before. The diagnostic criteria for Migraine without aura:

▌ Headache lasting four to seventy-two hours (untreated or treated unsuccessfully)

▌ The headache has at least two of the following characteristics:
- *unilateral (on one side) location*
- *pulsating quality*
- *moderate to severe intensity of pain*
- *pain aggravated by routine physical activity.*

▌ During the headache, at least one of the following:
- *nausea and/or vomiting*
- *phonophobia (sensitivity to sound) or photophobia (sensitivity to light)*

Migraine with Aura

EXAMPLE CASE: *Dawn's first indication of a Migraine attack is generally an aura symptom called olfactory hallucination. She smells smoke where there is none and has often searched her house looking for a fire. She also has visual aura symptoms she describes as zig-zag lines in her vision and sparks when she closes her eyes (scintillation). Although her auras were frightening to her at first, she says now she's glad she gets them with many of her Migraines because they give her the opportunity to take her medications earlier and possibly avoid the worst part of the Migraine attack. If she takes her triptan medication at the first aura symptoms, it will often abort the Migraine either before the head pain begins or before it becomes severe. Even if the triptan isn't that successful, the use of triptans has changed her treatment and life significantly. Before triptans were available, Dawn would take pain and nausea medications and retreat to her bed, sometimes for two or three days at a time. Preventive medications have also done a great deal to help Dawn. Not only does she experience fewer Migraine attacks, but triptans work better and more quickly than before.*

Previously called "classic Migraine." The most common scenario for Migraineurs diagnosed with Migraine with aura is that they're also diagnosed with Migraine without aura, since very, very few Migraineurs experience the aura phase with every Migraine. The diagnostic criteria for Migraine with aura:

▪ At least two known attacks
>   *and*
▪ Three of the following:
  • *one or more fully reversible aura symptoms*
  • *aura developing over more than four minutes*
  • *aura lasting less than sixty minutes*
  • *headache following aura within sixty minutes*

Abdominal Migraine

EXAMPLE CASE: *Eddie is a pretty typical six-year-old. His mother was at a loss when he started experiencing unexplained bouts of vomiting and abdominal pain accompanied by a refusal to eat and extreme paleness. After thoroughly examining Eddie, their pediatrician asked her if there was any family history of Migraine. Eddie's father has infrequent Migraine attacks, and his grandmother used to mention "sick headaches." He diagnosed Eddie with abdominal Migraine and prescribed medication for the nausea and vomiting. Now, when Eddie has a Migraine attack, his mother gives him his medication, and he's able to sleep for a while and wakes feeling much better.*

Abdominal Migraine is a form of Migraine seen mainly in children. It consists of abdominal pain, nausea, and vomiting. It was recognized as a form of Migraine disease as links were made to other family members having Migraines and children who had this disorder grew into adults with Migraine with and without aura. Most children who experience abdominal Migraine eventually develop Migraine with aura and/or Migraine without aura. The diagnostic criteria for abdominal Migraine are at least five attacks meeting the following:

▌ Attacks of abdominal pain lasting one to seventy-two hours (untreated or treated unsuccessfully)

▌ Abdominal pain with all of the following characteristics:
  • *midline location, periumbilical (around the navel), or poorly localized*
  • *dull or "just sore" quality*
  • *moderate or severe intensity*

▌ During abdominal pain, at least two of the following:
  • *anorexia (suppression of appetite)*
  • *nausea*
  • *vomiting*
  • *pallor (paleness)*

Familial Hemiplegic Migraine (FHM) and Sporadic Hemiplegic Migraine (SHM)

EXAMPLE CASE #1: *Frank has been diagnosed with familial hemiplegic Migraine since his grandfather and mother both experienced what are now thought to have been hemiplegic Migraines. His auras seldom last less than several hours and often last a couple of days. He takes antinausea medication as soon as his aura begins to control the nausea and vomiting that would otherwise accompany the attack. He experiences moderate to severe photophobia (sensitivity to light), but no phonophobia (sensitivity to sound). He also becomes very un-*

steady and has trouble walking well (ataxia). Usually, within thirty to sixty minutes of the onset of his head pain, hemiplegia (one-sided paralysis) sets in. Since triptans and ergotamines are contraindicated, he takes pain medications and tries to rest until the attacks pass. Frank reports that learning about this form of Migraine has been one of his best forms of treatment, because the knowledge has removed much of his apprehension, which allows him to rest better and allow the attack to run its course and pass.

EXAMPLE CASE #2: *Georgia has a family history of Migraine disease, but not hemiplegic Migraine. Therefore, her diagnosis is sporadic hemiplegic Migraine (SHM). When she had her first SHM, she went to the emergency room and was hospitalized because the doctor thought she was having a stroke. She'd had an aura for approximately thirty-six hours that had included aphasia (difficulty finding the right words to speak). Suddenly, one side of her body was paralyzed. By the time her family got her to the ER, she was experiencing severe head pain, nausea, and phonophobia. She was also running a fever. The doctor was concerned not only about the possibility of a stroke, but also about the possibility of meningitis. He ordered an MRI and lumbar puncture (spinal tap), then contacted the neurologist on call. Until that time, Georgia didn't have a neurologist on her medical team. The neurologist who was called in wasn't very familiar with forms of Migraine, and he didn't associate her symptoms with Migraine disease. He admitted her for observation and ordered pain medication for her. Luckily, when the test results didn't yield a diagnosis, he consulted a colleague who was able to arrive at a diagnosis and treatment plan for Georgia.*

Familial hemiplegic Migraine (FHM) and sporadic hemiplegic Migraine (SHM) sometimes begin in childhood and cease during adult years. Diagnosing FHM and SHM can be difficult, as the symptoms are also indicative of vascular (blood vessel) disease and can be thought to be indicative of stroke, epilepsy, or other conditions. A full neurological workup and careful review of medical history and symptoms are necessary to rule out other causes and confirm a diagnosis of FHM or SHM. Family medical history is especially helpful in diagnosing FHM. FHM and SHM share the same symptoms, which will vary among different Migraineurs. The difference between the two is that FHM can be traced back in the family history and has been linked to mutations of specific genes on chromosomes 1 and 19. SHM is FHM without the familial connection and that particular genetic mutation. Proper diagnosis of FHM and SHM is especially important because common Migraine-specific medications such as the triptans and ergotamines should not be prescribed for Migraineurs with hemiplegic Migraine. Migraineurs with hemiplegic Migraine should give special consideration to wearing some kind of medical identification at all times, since an attack can lead to impaired consciousness and an inability to speak. Medical identification can save valuable time in an emergency and assure that proper treatment is received far more quickly. Estimates of the frequency of hemiplegic Migraine vary from 4 to 30 percent of cases of Migraine. Symptoms of FHM and SHM include:

- episodes of prolonged aura (up to several days or weeks)
- hemiplegia (paralysis on one side of the body)
- fever
- meningismus (symptoms of meningitis without the actual illness and accompanying inflammation)
- impaired consciousness ranging from confusion to profound coma

▌ headache, which may begin before the hemiplegia or be absent

▌ ataxia (incoordination and unsteadiness due to the brain's failure to regulate the body's posture and regulate the strength and direction of limb movements)

▌ the onset of the hemiplegia may be sudden and simulate a stroke

▌ nausea and/or vomiting

▌ phonophobia (sensitivity to sound) and/or photophobia (sensitivity to light)

Basilar-Type Migraine

EXAMPLE CASE: *Heather was terrified the first time she experienced a basilar-type Migraine (BTM). She experienced terrible vertigo and bilateral paresthesias (abnormal or unpleasant sensation often described as numbness or a prickly, stinging, or burning feeling). During her aura, she developed tinnitus (ringing, hissing, or buzzing sound in the ears), vertigo, ataxia (incoordination and unsteadiness), and diplopia (double vision), and her level of consciousness declined, leaving her feeling "half here." Just as the diplopia cleared, she was even more terrified not to be able to see at all for a while. She describes that aura as a "horror show carnival ride," saying that one symptom would clear up only to be replaced almost immediately by another. Shortly, the head pain began and escalated to a fairly severe level. Since she had never experienced all these symptoms before, Heather called her doctor and was told to come in immediately. Fortunately, Heather's doctor recognized her BTM and knew how to treat it. Like hemiplegic Migraine, BTM should not be treated with triptans or ergotamines. So Heather can be sure she's not given these medications if she's unable to speak for herself, she now wears a Medic Alert bracelet.*

A basilar-type migraine (previously called basilar-artery Migraine or basilar Migraine) is a Migraine that has aura symptoms originating from the brain stem and/or affecting both hemispheres of the brain at the same time, but with no motor weakness. Many Migraineurs who have BTM also report Migraine with typical aura. The aura of BTM can include temporary blindness, which is one reason they can be quite terrifying. However, BTM is really Migraine with aura localized to the brain stem. Still, because of that localization, Migraine-specific medications such as the triptans and ergotamines are contraindicated for BTM. Once again, I highly recommend that Migraineurs who experience BTM wear some kind of medical identification at all times.

Diagnosis of BTM requires at least two attacks meeting the following criteria:

▌ Aura consisting of at least two of the following fully reversible symptoms, but no motor weakness:
- *dysarthria (impairments or clumsiness in the speaking of words due to diseases that affect the oral, lingual, or pharyngeal muscles)*
- *vertigo (sensation of moving around in space)*
- *tinnitus (ringing, hissing, or buzzing sound in the ears)*
- *hypacusia (impaired hearing)*
- *diplopia (double vision)*
- *visual symptoms simultaneously in both temporal and nasal fields of both eyes*
- *ataxia (incoordination and unsteadiness)*
- *decreased level of consciousness*
- *simultaneously bilateral (on both sides) paresthesias (ab-*

normal or unpleasant sensation often described as numbness or a prickly, stinging, or burning feeling)

▌ At least one of the following:
  - *at least one aura symptom develops gradually over five or more minutes and/or different aura symptoms occur in succession over five or more minutes*
  - *each aura symptom lasts between five and sixty minutes*

▌ Headache meeting the criteria for Migraine without aura begins during the aura or follows aura within sixty minutes

Retinal Migraine

EXAMPLE CASE #1: *Irene thought she had a horrible vision problem and, in fact, feared losing her vision. She had "spells" of what she described as "the strangest, scariest vision things followed by no vision at all in one eye." When she describes these spells in greater detail, we find that she experiences seeing twinkling lights of different brightness (scintillation), followed by small blank spots in her vision (scotoma). The scotoma then blend into total vision loss in one eye. The visual symptoms are quickly followed by head pain that matches the criteria for Migraine without aura—head pain, phonophobia (sensitivity to sound), and extreme nausea. It's important to note that her vision returns to normal after her Migraine attack and that all vision tests are normal (other than her usual myopia) between Migraine attacks.*

EXAMPLE CASE #2: *Jason's symptoms are much like Irene's with one major exception—he seldom experiences the headache phase. Still, his diagnosis is the same, retinal Migraine. To this may be added the descriptive (not diagnostic) term* acephalgic, *which simply means "without head pain." Thus, most of Jason's are acephalgic retinal Migraine attacks.*

INTERESTING NOTE: *Jason's original diagnosis was "ocular Migraine." If we adhere to the International Headache Society classifications, there is no diagnosis of "ocular Migraine." It's understandable that his ophthalmologist used the term, since when he skips the headache phase, all his symptoms are visual. The problem with using a "descriptive diagnosis" as opposed to one from the accepted listing is that other doctors can't be sure exactly what the original physician intended.*

Retinal Migraine is a form of Migraine characterized by repeated attacks of monocular (in one eye) visual disturbance, including scintillations (perception of twinkling light of varying intensity), scotoma (area or areas of decreased or lost vision), or blindness along with Migraine without aura. It's important that other causes of transient one-eyed blindness be ruled out before diagnosing with retinal Migraine. Once other possible causes are ruled out, diagnosis of retinal Migraine requires at least two attacks meeting the following criteria:

▌ Fully reversible monocular visual phenomena (such as scintillations, scotoma, or blindness) confirmed by examination during an attack or (after proper instruction) by the patient's drawing of a monocular field defect during an attack.
Plain English version: Experiencing twinkling lights of varying intensity (scintillations), areas of decreased or lost vision (scotoma), or other visual phenomena in one eye only (monocular) during an attack. Fully reversible means that these symptoms end when the Migraine attack ends.

The symptoms need to be confirmed by an examination during an attack or by the patient, at a later time, drawing what was seen.

▌ Headache fulfilling criteria for Migraine without aura begins during the visual symptoms and/or follows them within sixty minutes

▌ Normal examination by an ophthalmologist between attacks

Chronic Migraine

EXAMPLE CASE: *Kathy has had Migraine attacks for approximately ten years. In the last two years, she has developed chronic Migraine and experiences Migraine attacks at least four days a week, sometimes more. (Been there, done that, burned the T-shirt! I'm keeping my fingers crossed for you, Kathy!) She experiences both Migraine with aura and Migraine without aura, which is common. To avoid rebound, her doctor recommends that she use triptans the first two or three days of a week that she has Migraines, then she can use pain and antinausea meds two more days that week if she needs to. The goal is to abort as many of her Migraine attacks as possible, relieve the pain of those they can't abort without risking triptan rebound, and avoid analgesic rebound while trying to find an effective preventive regimen for her. Ten years ago, Kathy's case would have seemed much more discouraging. Today, there are so many preventive medications and combinations of them that effective preventive regimens can be found for most Migraineurs.*

Chronic Migraine is Migraine with headache phase occurring fifteen or more days per month for more than three months when there is no rebound headache, aka medication overuse headache. It is sometimes called "transformed Migraine." Attacks need to meet these diagnostic criteria:

▮ Headache has at least two of the following characteristics:
- *unilateral (on one side) location*
- *pulsating (throbbing with the pulse) quality*
- *moderate or severe pain intensity*
- *aggravation by or causing avoidance of routine physical activity (such as walking or climbing stairs)*

▮ During headache at least one of the following:
- *nausea and/or vomiting*
- *photophobia (sensitivity to light) and phonophobia (sensitivity to sound)*

Status Migrainous

Status Migrainous is a Migraine attack with a debilitating headache that lasts more than seventy-two hours. When determining the seventy-two-hour duration, neither interruption during sleep nor short-lasting relief due to medication counts as a break in the seventy-two hours.

This is where it's important to remember what I said earlier about the cause of Migraine. The key part of that when discussing status Migrainous is, "The headache of a Migraine attack, if there is one, is from sensory impulses transmitted by the nerves from these *inflamed blood vessels* and surrounding tissues." When we're experiencing headache during a Migraine, blood vessels in our brains are inflamed. A goal of Migraine treatment is to return those blood vessels to normal size as soon as possible. When they're inflamed for long periods of time, our risk of stroke increases.

This is a time when medical treatment should be sought. If it's a weekend or after hours, or your doctor isn't in for another reason, go to the emergency room.

ABI'S STORY

Abi was a vibrant young woman, recently engaged and full of plans for her life. The main problem in her life was her Migraines. They were brutal and sometimes lasted for days.

One Wednesday evening, we were talking in my About. com chat room with a small group. Abi had had a Migraine for five days. I pleaded with her to ask her mother to take her to the emergency room. She said she couldn't because her parents had accused her of faking her Migraines for attention. We talked awhile longer, then Abi logged off to try to sleep.

On Friday, I got an e-mail from Abi's fiancé, telling me that she'd had a stroke that day and was in the hospital. The doctor said quite plainly that the extended Migraine had caused the stroke. Her fiancé asked that I let Abi's "Migraine family" know and that we pray for her.

We were all so happy when Abi appeared to recover from the stroke and went home from the hospital. About a week later, however, Abi had another Migraine. She treated it immediately but had another stroke within hours of the beginning of the Migraine. This time, she didn't survive the stroke. She passed away just days short of her twenty-second birthday.

Whether Abi had a premonition that she'd have another stroke, was just fearful of them, or was just writing her feelings, we'll never know, but during the time between her strokes, she wrote a letter to me in her journal. Her fiancé copied it into an e-mail and sent it to me. Part of it said, "Can you do me a favor? Could you please help others understand about Migraine, and that getting immediate treatment is important?"

There you have it. That's Abi's story. I honor her last request of me by sharing her story with you.

Migraine Disease and Stroke Risk

There has been some debate and a bit of controversy surrounding Migraine disease and stroke risk for some time now. When I began researching the field of headache and Migraine, I came across some study results published in medical journals that showed an increased risk of stroke for people with Migraine disease. These studies never got much attention, and many people tended to dismiss the concept that just having the disease could present an increased risk of stroke. My opinion on the subject was that although the risk wasn't significant enough to be especially worrisome, it was something Migraineurs should know and a darned good reason for us to do what we could in our lifestyles to minimize stroke risk. In late 2004, researchers compiled the results of fourteen studies on Migraine disease and stroke risk. The result of their analysis:

- The average risk of stroke for all Migraineurs is 2.16 times that of people without Migraine.
- Adding oral contraceptives increases the risk of stroke by approximately 8 times.

Now, before you let those figures alarm you too much, we need to put them in context. The average stroke prevalence in women in the general population is 9 per 100,000, which represents absolute risk. If patients with Migraine have an average of 2.16 times greater risk, that's about 20 per 100,000, still a very low absolute risk. On oral contraceptives, the absolute risk is about 75 per 100,000.

This information is not reason for panic or excessive worrying. It's wise for everyone to discuss lifestyle and stroke risk with his or her doctors. This is another example of the patient retaining control. Many stroke risks can be lessened with lifestyle changes. The doctors I've spoken with say the biggest stroke risk of all is smoking.

If you're using oral contraceptives, talk to your doctor about the dose of estrogen in them. Lowering the dose of estrogen in the pill probably reduces much of the stroke risk.

Summary

As you can see, Migraine diagnoses can be confusing. The International Headache Society "International Classification of Headache Disorders" is accepted as the standard for classification by many doctors. However, there are still doctors who don't use it and give other Migraine diagnoses. This can make things terribly confusing. For example, people will come to my forums and say they have "ocular Migraines." They're looking for people with the same kind of Migraine to talk with. In some cases, given their symptoms, their attacks sound like retinal Migraines; in some cases, they sound like Migraine with aura. If for some reason these Migraineurs need to go to another doctor, that doctor isn't going to be told much by their diagnosis, either. If you're given a Migraine diagnosis, ask if it's one from the IHS classification. That will be helpful to you if you ever need to seek treatment when on vacation or away from home for another reason.

Now that we've gone through the medical part of this chapter, how about some lighter information? It's interesting to note some of the famous Migraineurs through history and today. In some cases, you can see how their Migraines may well have affected their work and their places in history:

- Lewis Carroll, author of *Alice's Adventures in Wonderland* and *Through the Looking-Glass, and What Alice Found There*
- Virginia Woolf
- Cervantes

- Vincent van Gogh
- Claude Monet
- Georges Seurat
- Thomas Jefferson
- Julius Caesar
- Ulysses S. Grant
- Robert E. Lee
- Mary Todd Lincoln
- Sigmund Freud
- Elizabeth Taylor
- Lee Grant
- Loretta Lynn
- Star Jones
- Whoopi Goldberg
- Courtney Thorne-Smith
- Kareem Abdul-Jabbar
- Scotty Pippen
- Monica Seles
- Elvis Presley! Elvis is a truly sad tale of Migraine disease. In the United States in the 1970s, there were still many people who considered Migraines to be a psychosomatic illness. Thus, "the King" never disclosed that he was a Migraineur. Several years ago, Michael John Coleman, executive director of MAGNUM, the National Migraine Association, was able to locate and interview Dr. George Nichopoulos, Elvis's personal physician. Some of you may remember that Elvis was hospitalized in 1973 for "headache and mild hypertension" and again in 1975 for "extensive eye exam." Dr. Nichopoulos confirmed that both hospitalizations were Migraine related and that Elvis suffered from chronic Migraine. Information leaked from his autopsy indicated that Elvis had Demerol, propranolol, LSD, and antiemetics in his bloodstream at the time of his death. Since his Migraine

disease had been kept secret, nobody understood that those medications did not indicate drug abuse or addiction. DHE (dihydroergotamine), a Migraine abortive medication, will show up in a blood test as LSD, an ergot alkaloid that is structurally related to LSD. Elvis was taking propranolol as a Migraine preventive. DHE can be used only a certain number of times a month, so Elvis used Demerol for his Migraines when he couldn't take DHE. Antiemetics are very frequently prescribed for Migraineurs. Thus, thanks to the closed minds of society, he was labeled a drug abuser rather than a man with a neurological disease.

Now that we've established what Migraine disease is and the different types of Migraine, we'll cover triggers, treatments, and other issues in other chapters. Stay tuned.

6

Cluster Headaches

EXAMPLE CASE: *Bob will be headache-free for months, then be struck by a cycle of cluster headaches that occur several times daily for up to a week. The pain is unilateral (one-sided) and so severe that Bob describes it as feeling "like someone is driving a barbecue skewer into my eye." Along with the more than excruciating pain, he experiences ipsilateral (on the same side as the pain) lacrimation (tearing), rhinorrhea (runny nose), and eyelid edema (swelling). He is totally unable to lie down, but he paces the floor. After he's exhausted himself doing that, he can sometimes "rest" by bending a bit at the waist and leaning the affected side of his head against a wall. As he leans, putting more of his weight on his head, he says it will sometimes actually make the pain seem a tiny bit less. He confesses to having banged his head against that wall more than once. DHE and triptans do nothing to relieve Bob's headaches. Strong prescription pain relievers barely take the edge off the pain. He says he's glad each headache usually lasts less than an hour because he doesn't know how much longer he could stand the pain. Because each headache lasts less than an hour, emergency room treatment isn't really an option—the headache would be over before he was treated. Fortunately for his livelihood, Bob works for a company and supervisor willing to make accommodations for him. During a cluster cycle, they're very understanding if he closes himself in his office or stays home.*

Cluster headaches have been called "suicide headaches." They affect between 1 and 4 percent of the population and occur in men more often than women. For those who have experienced them, clusters are the most painful headache anyone can have. The pain has been described as "boring," "tearing," or "burning." Analogies also are used, such as "a hot poker in the eye" or feeling as if "the eye is being pushed out." Anyone who has ever had a cluster headache has no doubt what they are. It's no exaggeration to say that the pain and desperation of cluster headaches have actually led to suicides.

Cluster headaches have been known by many names throughout the years—migrainous neuralgia, histamine cephalagia, petrosal neuralgia, sphenopalatine neuralgia, Sluder's neuralgia, and Horton's headache, to name just a few. Its final designation came from the headache's pattern to cluster, in both number of headaches per day and number of days in an attack. One of the best descriptions of a cluster headache that I've seen comes from the middle of the eighteenth century and is published in *Headache in Clinical Practice* by Stephen Silberstein et al:

A healthy, robust man of middle age [was suffering from] troublesome pain which came on every day at the same hour at the same spot above the orbit of the left eye, where the nerve emerges from the opening of the frontal bone; after a short time the left eye began to redden and to overflow with tears; then he felt as if his eye was slowly forced out of its orbit with so much pain, that he nearly went mad. After a few hours all these evils ceased, and nothing in the eye appeared at all changed.

Cluster headaches are attacks of severe, strictly unilateral (one-sided) pain that is orbital (around the bony cavity that holds the eye), supraorbital (above the orbit), temporal (at the temple), or in any combination of these sites, lasting 15 to 180 minutes and occurring from once every other day to eight times a day. The attacks are associated with one or more of the following, all of which are ipsilateral (on the same side as the headache): conjunctival injection (the forcing of a fluid into the conjunctiva, the mucous membrane that lines the eyelids), lacrimation (tearing), nasal congestion, rhinorrhea (runny nose), forehead and facial sweating, miosis (abnormal contraction of the pupils), ptosis (drooping of the eyelid), and/or eyelid edema. Most people are restless or agitated during an attack and cannot lie down. A diagnosis of cluster headache requires at least five attacks fulfilling these criteria:

- Severe or very severe unilateral (one-sided) orbital (around the bony cavity that holds the eye), supraorbital (above the orbit), and/or temporal pain lasting 15 to 180 minutes if untreated
- Headache is accompanied by at least one of the following:
  - *ipsilateral (on the same side as the headache) conjunctival injection (the forcing of a fluid into the conjunctiva, the mucous membrane that lines the eyelids) and/or lacrimation (tearing)*
  - *ipsilateral nasal congestion and/or rhinorrhea (runny nose)*
  - *ipsilateral eyelid edema (swelling)*
  - *ipsilateral forehead and facial sweating*

- *ipsilateral miosis (contraction of the pupil) and/or ptosis (drooping eyelid)*
- *a sense of restlessness or agitation*
▌ Attacks have a frequency from one every other day to eight per day

Once the diagnosis of cluster headache is made, there are also two classifications within that diagnosis:

▌ *Episodic cluster headache:* Cluster headache attacks occurring in periods lasting seven days to one year, separated by pain-free periods lasting one month or longer.
▌ *Chronic cluster headache:* Cluster headache attacks occurring for more than one year without remission or with remissions lasting less than one month. Chronic cluster headaches may be chronic from the beginning or evolve from the episodic subtype. Some people may switch from chronic to episodic cluster headache.

The Cause of Cluster Headaches

Modern imaging technology is a wonderful thing; it has allowed us to learn so much more than we could have without it. PET (positron emission tomography) scans measure the activity of the brain. PET scans of patients done during cluster headaches show that the hypothalamus is activated during an attack. The pain is caused by activation of the trigeminal nerve, which is responsible for sensation to most of the head and around the eye. The eyelid edema (swelling), sweating, and rhinorrhea (runny nose) of a cluster headache come from activation of the parasympathetic nervous system. Cluster sufferers can exhibit a droopy eyelid and small pupil on the cluster side if there is swelling around the carotid artery behind the eye that damages the sympathetic nervous system.

Cluster Headaches Can Be Tricky

Especially before diagnosis, it can be difficult to tell the difference between a cluster headache and a Migraine attack. It doesn't help that it's not unusual for people to experience both clusters and Migraines and possibly tension headaches as well. Clusters may vary from Migraines is some notable ways:

- Unlike Migraine, cluster headaches do not have discernible phases (that is, prodrome, aura, headache, and postdrome). A cluster headache usually comes on without any warning; however, some individuals in a few studies have reported an aura or premonitory warning. Gastrointestinal symptoms are not usually reported with cluster headaches; although nausea has been reported in up to 40 percent of cases, vomiting is rare.
- Clusters, unlike Migraines, can be short in duration, anywhere from 15 to 180 minutes per attack, occurring several times a day over many days or weeks. Clusters can go into remission, giving the patient weeks, months, or even years of relief from attacks.
- During a cluster headache, it is more often very difficult to lie down, and people are known to pace the floor or keep moving in some other way. During a Migraine attack, movement most often worsens the pain, making it far preferable to lie down.
- Cluster headaches are more common in men than women. Interestingly, the estimated prevalence ratio has been

changing drastically over the years. By 1995, the ratio was estimated to be 2.1:1, far closer than in the past. Researchers theorize that women have long been misdiagnosed because cluster headaches were thought to be found so predominantly in men. Migraines are more common in women than men at a ratio of 4:1.

▋ Cluster headaches are far less common, occurring in 0.4 percent of the population. Migraine occurs in 12 percent of the population.

This gives us a good foundation on cluster headaches. We'll be discussing triggers, treatment, and more in later chapters.

7

Rebound, aka Medication Overuse Headaches

EXAMPLE CASE: *Ronnie's doctor had prescribed aceta-*
minophen with hydrocodone (Vicodin) for her Migraine at-
tacks. The instructions on the label read, "One tablet every
six hours as needed for headache." Ronnie was very careful
not to take the medication any more frequently than directed.
When her Migraine was severe enough that she thought she
might lose track of time, she'd write down the time she
took the medication and start a stopwatch. Following a pe-
riod of frequent Migraine attacks, Ronnie was experiencing
headaches daily, but she realized they were headaches, not Mi-
graine attacks. The pain was bilateral (on both sides) and
wasn't made worse by bending over, and she didn't have any
other symptoms. She made an appointment with her doctor,
who said, "Oh, those are rebound headaches. You have to
stop taking all pain medication for them to stop."

They're called rebound headaches, analgesic rebound headaches,
or medication overuse headaches, but nobody ever told me about rebound headaches—ever. Now that I realize what I went through

with them a couple of times, I certainly wish someone had. The first time I came across any mention of rebound headaches was when I was doing research of my own for an article I was writing. As I thought back to some episodes when pain medications worked initially but I'd be in pain again the next day, I had one of those "light bulb moments," realizing that what I had experienced were rebound headaches. Luckily, I had always decided to quit taking the medications if I knew the headache was going to come back the next day anyway. After a while the pain stopped, but I never thought to associate it with the medication. After all, pain medications are supposed to relieve pain, not cause it. Right? Well, yes. That's certainly what a reasonable person expects.

So what are rebound headaches? They're headaches caused by the overuse of medications, mostly analgesics (pain relievers). Simplified, what happens is this: We get a headache or Migraine, and we take medication for it. If we take that medication more than two or three days a week, our bodies get used to it being there. Then, when we don't take it, our bodies do what it took to get us to take the medication in the first place, which is produce a headache.

Signs of Rebound Headache

- Increase in headache frequency
- Irresistible use of increasing amounts of the medication that brought on the rebound
- Failure of alternate medications to relieve the headache
- A new pattern of awakening with or developing a headache at the same time every day
- Predictable occurrence of headache within hours to days after the last dose of the rebound-causing medication
- Taking more or stronger medication, but getting less relief

What Medications Cause Rebound/Medication Overuse Headaches?

"What meds cause rebound?" is one of the questions I get most frequently. This is an area where it's taken a while to see a consensus begin to form among specialists in the field. Agreement was reached early on regarding analgesics and NSAIDs (nonsteroidal anti-inflammatory drugs) such as aspirin, acetaminophen, ibuprofen, naproxen sodium, ketoprofen, and compound medications containing them, as well as the abortive medication DHE (dihydroergotamine). The list has grown from there. Some doctors simplify things by saying "all analgesics." When you look at that phrase, you need to remember the definition of analgesic. An analgesic is any medication that relieves pain. That covers a lot of ground. In his book *Understanding Migraine and Other Headaches,* Dr. Stewart Tepper offers us his two-part list:

▌ **Over-the-counter medications**
- *Analgesics such as aspirin, acetaminophen, ibuprofen, and the like*
- *Mixed analgesics such as Excedrin, BC powder, and others*
- *Nasal decongestants such as pseudoephedrine (Sudafed)*
- *Antihistamines such as diphenhydramine (Benadryl) and dimenhydrinate*
- *Mixed cold and allergy medications such as Sinutab, Dimetapp, and so forth*
- *Sleeping medications*
- *Caffeine*

▌ **Prescription medications**
- *Analgesics such as tramadol, codeine, hydrocodone, morphine, and methadone*
- *NSAIDs such as ibuprofen, naproxen, and ketorolac*

- *Tranquilizers such as butalbital (found in Fiorinal and Fioricet), diazepam, and lorazepam*
- *Ergots, including DHE, Migranal, and others*
- *Triptans: all*

Along with the obvious fact that we have a headache, rebound headaches present us with other problems, some of which can extend beyond our head pain to our general health:

▌ If you're trying to find an effective preventive regimen, you can pretty much forget about that until the rebound cycle is broken. Our preventives usually won't work when we're in rebound. **Anecdote:** A young woman recently told me that she was in a deep rebound cycle, but her doctor told her not to worry about that just yet. He prescribed a preventive medication and told her the rebound headaches would stop once the preventive took effect. Sigh. I think not.

▌ The only medication that's going to seem to give adequate relief from rebound headache is the medication that caused the rebound in the first place. Sometimes others will give limited relief for a short period of time.

▌ Some of the medications often prescribed for headache and Migraine are butalbital compounds such as Fioricet, Fiorinal, Esgic, Phrenilin, and others. There are variations on the compounds, but they all have butalbital, which is a barbiturate, along with either aspirin or acetaminophen. Some also have caffeine. These meds present a double or even triple rebound problem—the aspirin or acetaminophen, the butalbital, and possibly caffeine. The butalbital can present special problems, because depending on the amount the person has been taking, it can cause seizures if withdrawn too abruptly.

▌ We have to consider possible future health care needs. We don't know what the future holds. We may have a time when, owing to illness, disease, or surgery, we need effective pain management. Building a tolerance to pain meds now is something we could well regret later.

▌ Increasingly, cases of overdose and toxicity from even over-the-counter medications are being reported:

- *In June 2003, a seventeen-year-old girl in Texas died after taking 500-mg tablets of acetaminophen for a Migraine. The acetaminophen caused her liver and kidneys to fail. The young woman wasn't trying to hurt herself. I recently received an e-mail from the young woman's mother, who is trying to find a way to make more people aware of the dangers of taking too much acetaminophen. She gave me permission to share that letter with you:*

KELLIE'S STORY

Teri,

I wanted to write explaining to you the dangers of acetaminophen and ask why no one does anything to stop this. You see, I HAD a beautiful daughter named Kellie. She, as I do, suffered with Migraines, but she wouldn't take anything stronger than Tylenol.

On the morning of June 26, 2003, Kellie got a Migraine around 3:00 a.m., so she took some Tylenol. She vomited, so she took more, not realizing it had already been digested. This happened three or four more times. She ended up taking up to 20 in a 16-hour period. Around 4:00 p.m., she started having severe stomach pain. I took her to the hospital then. At the hospital, they took blood, started the "antidote," and gave her some "charcoal stuff," which she threw up. She said, "Mom, I'm sorry. I tried to keep it down." I told her, "It's OK, don't worry about it."

She said, "I thought it was OK, Mom. It was only Tylenol." I said, "It's OK, Kel." I had no idea what was to come of it. I figured she'd be OK. WRONG!!! The doctor came in and told me that, at that point, Kellie had an 80 percent chance of dying. You could have blown me over with a feather. The doctor told me, "You need to call whoever you need to. She might not make it through the night." I was horrified and in shock. I couldn't understand why he was saying that and went into denial mode. I called my husband and told him to get there as fast as possible. He argued with me; he was in shock, too.

The next day, Kellie started going into convulsions, and they transferred her to a hospital where they could do transplants. The Tylenol had started to shut her liver down. There is no liver machine; transplant was her only chance. They put her on the "list" as #1, but there wasn't a liver available. They put her into a medically induced coma to "lessen the stress on the organs," we were told. We had called our son, who lived in Georgia, and he immediately flew out here. Kellie was his only sister. He loved her very much. By the time he got here, she was in the coma. On June 25, Kellie's kidneys shut down. On June 27, the doctors put a screw into Kellie's brain to monitor the fluid; they then found out that she started getting water on the brain. On June 28, the doctors told us she was brain-dead. We as a family had to make a decision to keep her alive as a vegetable or let her go. She wouldn't know who she was or who we were. The only part of her brain that was still functioning at that time was the part that was keeping her organs going. We all agreed Kellie would not want to live like that, for that is not living. We then made the decision for Kellie to be a donor, in hopes of saving someone else. Her heart was still good and her eyes and other parts, but unfortunately she developed an infection and no organs could be used. I truly believe if Kellie had gotten a liver she would be with us now. That's why I believe strongly in organ donation. Livers

*do not age. Unless they're damaged, they regenerate them-
selves, and without a liver machine, a transplant is the only
hope of survival.*

*Without even being able to say, "good-bye," or "I love
you," we watched her slowly die as the machines slowly shut
down. On June 28, 2003, at 6:00 p.m., Kellie was pro-
nounced dead.*

*Please get this across to your readers in hope no one else
has to live through a hell like this.*

Thank you,

Jodie

- In 2003, the most recent year for which there are official
  statistics, there were 40,833 accidental acetaminophen
  overdoses and 20,113 intentional overdoses. Of all the
  overdoses, 147 of them were fatal.

Breaking the Rebound Cycle

If we've accidentally taken medications a couple of days more than
we should have and have gotten into rebound that way, we can often handle it ourselves by not taking more of that medication or any
other pain medication for several days or a bit longer. Usually, however, people get into a rebound cycle without realizing it. Getting
our doctor's help is the best place to start. Depending on what medication has caused the problem, there may be different options.
Sometimes the best option a doctor can offer us really is just to stop
pain meds and get through it. Giving us something else for pain
won't help. In some situations, they may be able to prescribe another type of medication to help us withdraw from the problem
medication.

Sometimes hospitalization for getting the problem medication out of our system is the best solution. If this is what your doctor suggests, please don't let it upset you. It doesn't mean you're a "drug addict" or that your doctor is saying you are. It just means that's the method your doctor thinks is best for your health. For example, Dr. Elizabeth Loder and Dr. David Biondi in Boston have developed an inpatient method for helping patients who are suffering butalbital compound rebound. With their method, the patients run no risk of seizure and are kept comfortable while the butalbital works its way out of their system. At the same time, they work with the patients on education, alternative pain control strategies, and other areas so they are better prepared to leave the hospital.

When you are working with a doctor to plan a way out of rebound, it's also important to plan ahead with preventive medications, abortive medications, and other strategies to address the situation that caused the meds (that caused the rebound) to be taken in the first place. Unless you do that, the problem that led to rebound is still there, and believe me, that is not good. Again, been there, done that, burned the T-shirt.

But My Head Hurts Every Day. What Do I Do?

If we could come up with one simple answer to that, we could win the Nobel Prize, have the money to be sure everyone had good health care, and retire very contented people. That's not to say there's no answer, but there's no one simple answer.

We can probably all agree that the best thing for dealing with daily headaches would be effective trigger management and preventive therapies so that our heads didn't hurt frequently enough for rebound to occur. Right? Let me offer you a bit of hope on that front. Enough progress has been made in recent years that effective preventive regimens can be found for at least 95–98 percent of people with chronic headaches and Migraine disease. For those of you my age, let's just say "mature readers," you know how much progress that is. Some of you younger readers may not realize how significant a leap that is. If you haven't had headaches or Migraines very long, you may not even remember a time when triptans such as Imitrex and Maxalt weren't available to people with Migraines and cluster headaches. Imitrex was the first of those drugs, introduced in the U.S. market in 1992.

For those of us who need pain relief more than two or three days a week, the next option is working with our doctors to find a treatment plan that involves two different classes of medications so we can use one of them for two or three days a week and the other one for two or three days a week. Much of this depends on the doctor, but there are such treatment plans. In most cases, doctors will want to continue to work on finding effective preventive treatments so the need for pain meds can be reduced.

> Your doctor should talk about both preventives to reduce the frequency of your Migraines and different classes of medication for acute Migraine treatment to help avoid rebound. If not, ask. These are your keys to staying free of rebound.

8

Other Headache Disorders

There are many, many different headache disorders, not to mention headaches caused by other illnesses. To try to list and describe them all here would be both impossible and pointless. We've already covered the most common disorders. Here, we'll spend some time on the basics of other headache disorders common enough that you may encounter them or know someone who does.

Coital (Sexual) Headache

Coital headache is divided into two subtypes: preorgasmic and orgasmic. Both subtypes are headache precipitated by sexual activity. They generally begin as a dull bilateral (on both sides) ache as sexual excitement increases and suddenly become intense at or immediately following orgasm. For preorgasmic headache, the diagnostic criteria require both of the following:

■ Dull ache in the head and neck associated with neck and/or jaw muscle contraction

▪ Occurs during sexual activity and increases with sexual excitement

The diagnostic criteria for orgasmic headache require both of the following:

▪ Sudden, severe headache sometimes described as "explosive"
▪ Occurs at orgasm

Before confirming a diagnosis of this type of headache, it is essential to rule out subarachnoid hemorrhage and arterial dissection with an imaging study.

Interesting note: We've all heard, and probably laughed about, the statement, "Not tonight, dear. I have a headache." Now I've introduced you to coital headache. Interestingly enough, for some Migraineurs, orgasm can actually have the opposite effect. Some Migraineurs find that, especially when achieved early in the attack, an orgasm can actually abort a Migraine attack. It's true! I promise. It doesn't work for every Migraineur, but it absolutely does work for some.

Exertional Headache

EXAMPLE CASE #1: *Alexander likes to work out to stay in shape. He jogs daily, does longer runs on weekends, and works out at a gym three times a week. When he first wrote to me, it was because he had started having severe headaches following his sessions at the gym. They'd strike suddenly and last at least two hours. Over-the-counter pain relievers only partly relieved the pain. After consulting his doctor, he let me know that he'd been diagnosed with exertional headaches. His doctor prescribed a medication for him to take before going to the gym. It successfully prevents those exertional headaches, allowing Alexander to continue his active and healthy lifestyle.*

Exertional headaches are any headache brought on by any form of exercise. Diagnosis criteria from the IHS for exertional headache are

▌ Pulsating headache fulfilling both of the following:
  • *duration of 5 minutes to 48 hours*
  • *brought on by and occurring only during or after physical exertion*

As with coital headache, before you confirm a diagnosis of this type of headache, it is essential to rule out subarachnoid hemorrhage and arterial dissection with an imaging study.

Hemicrania Continua

EXAMPLE CASE: *Beth had been suffering with a constant unilateral (one-sided) headache for over a year when I first met her. Over a year without a single pain-free moment! There were what she called flare-ups when the pain would escalate and she would experience other symptoms, including lacrimation (tearing) and rhinorrhea (runny nose) on the same side as her headache. Her family doctor had referred her to two neurologists, both of whom had diagnosed her with chronic Migraine without aura but had been unable to find anything to give her any relief. Her MRI results had been negative. She was at the end of her rope and wasn't sure there was even enough rope left to tie a good knot. While she held on, we located a good headache specialist and got her an appointment. At her first appointment, the specialist reviewed her medical history, the medical records and MRI films she had taken with her, and her symptoms. He conducted a neurological examination and found all to be normal—except for her pain. He told her it was his opinion that she had hemicrania continua and that trying indomethacin should confirm the diagnosis. She had a prescription for indomethacin filled on her way home and began taking it. A week later, she was pain-free for the first time in eighteen months.*

Hemicrania continua is a persistent, strictly unilateral (one-sided) headache that is always responsive to indomethacin. Hemicrania continua is usually unremitting, but rare cases of remission are reported. A diagnosis of hemicrania continua requires meeting the following IHS criteria:

▌ Headache for more than three months fulfilling the following:
  - *All of the following characteristics:*
    - unilateral (one-sided) pain without side shift (changing sides)
    - daily and continuous, without pain-free period
    - moderate intensity, but with exacerbations of severe pain
  - *At least one of the following features occurring during exacerbations and on the same side as the pain:*
    - conjunctival injection (forcing of a fluid into the conjunctiva, the mucous membrane that lines the eyelids) and/or lacrimation (tearing)
    - nasal congestion and/or rhinorrhea (runny nose)

- ptosis (drooping of the eyelid) and/or miosis (abnormal contraction of the pupils)
- *Complete response to therapeutic doses of indomethacin*

Ice Pick Headache

Ice pick headaches have been described in varying ways. Here are some descriptions that have been written to me:

- ▌ "In the beginning, when I began having migraines, I suffered a sudden slash of pain, very intense and quick on the right side of my head. It started at one point and webbed out to what felt like a inch in length. I had never felt this type of pain, and it scared me."
- ▌ "They are intense, sharp, stabbing pains about your skull, as if you were being stabbed with an ice pick."
- ▌ "I was awakened at 3:00 a.m. by excruciating, stabbing pains on the top right front of my head, kind of behind the eye. It lasted about thirty seconds."
- ▌ "I get those types of stabbing pains, I have no clue as to what is causing it. I get them all over my head. They can last for a few seconds to a few minutes. I started noticing them after my migraines started to get to where they were coming about three to four days a week."
- ▌ "I have these very sudden, sharp pains in my head on a daily basis. It feels as if I'm being stabbed in the head."

Under the International Headache Society's criteria, the official name for them is "primary stabbing headache." The IHS description is: "Transient and localized stabs of pain in the head that occur spontaneously in the absence of organic disease of underlying structures or of the cranial nerves." Diagnosis of ice pick headache requires head pain occurring as a single stab or a series of stabs and fulfilling these criteria:

▌ exclusively or predominantly felt in the distribution of the first division of the trigeminal nerve (orbit, temple, and parietal area)
▌ stabs last for up to a few seconds and recur with irregular frequency ranging from one to many per day
▌ no accompanying symptoms

Other terms that have been used are idiopathic stabbing headache jabs and jolts, ophthalmodynia, and periodica. Ice pick headache is probably the most commonly used term because it's the most descriptive.

Although people who experience ice pick headaches are usually those who have Migraine disease or another head pain disorder, ice pick headaches generally occur by themselves rather than during a Migraine attack or headache. Typically they occur a few times a day at most. Occasionally, however, they occur frequently through the day, requiring treatment. The major problem with treatment, of course, is that the pain is so brief, if it's not treated until it occurs, it's gone before the patient can even take medication. In those rare cases where it does need treatment, preventive treatment with indomethacin (Indocin) usually works.

In an article published in *Current Pain and Headache Reports,* Dr. Todd Rozen summarized the situation of people with ice pick headaches quite succinctly:

The short-lasting headache syndromes are unique based on their short duration of pain and their associated symptoms. Physicians need to be knowledgeable about these syndromes because each has its own distinct treatment and if the diagno-

sis is missed, the patient can be burdened with extreme headache-related disability.

Ice pick headaches occur in up to 40 percent of Migraineurs, often located in or near the usual location of their Migraines. They can occur at any time of day or even wake people from sleep. Those who do need to use indomethacin for prevention should remember that it is a nonsteroidal anti-inflammatory drug and has the potential side effects typically associated with NSAIDs. Those potential side effects include heartburn, nausea, gastroesophageal reflux and bleeding problems, and gastric ulcers. In rare cases, indomethacin can cause eye problems. Thus, annual examinations by an ophthalmologist are recommended for anyone taking it on a regular basis.

If you're experiencing what you think may be ice pick headaches, please don't just assume that's what they are. Log them in your diary and go see your doctor. As with any other head pain, there can be too many possible causes to guess. A doctor's diagnosis is vital.

Post-Traumatic Headache

SAMPLE CASE #1: *Patti was injured at work when a large sheet of glass that was being moved overhead fell and hit her. It was just weeks before her wedding, and she was more concerned about the cuts she suffered than the headache she had. She thought the headache would go away in a day or two. Thanks to luck, a good plastic surgeon, and some makeup, the cuts were all but invisible on their wedding day, but Patti was in a lot of pain with the headache that persisted, and her new husband postponed their honeymoon. The headache pain was moderate, not severe, but its persistence concerned them both. It was bilateral, somewhat like a tension-type headache. It also soon became apparent that Patti's forgetfulness, which they had been attributing to prewedding jitters, was possibly connected to the headaches. Unable to help Patti achieve any significant relief, her family doctor and neurologist helped her find a headache specialist to treat her. At the three-month mark, the specialist diagnosed her with chronic post-traumatic headache. A combination of preventive medications helped reduce the frequency of her headaches, allowing her to need acute treatment only two or three days a week, which avoided rebound issues. After about eighteen months, Patti's headache frequency began to decrease dramatically. Eventually she was able to taper off the preventive medications, and the headaches have stopped.*

SAMPLE CASE #2: *Randy was injured in a skiing accident. He took quite a tumble and hit his head on a tree. (Despite his jokes, the tree was harder than his head.) He had a mild concussion, so he was kept in the hospital overnight for observation, then discharged. In a couple of weeks, he had recovered and quickly dismissed the incident. Approximately five years later, he began having severe throbbing headaches accompanied by nausea and photophobia (sensitivity to light). His doctor ordered an MRI, which was negative. They considered Migraine disease, but Randy exhibits no Migraine symptoms other than photophobia. His headaches are unusual for Migraine because they are bilateral and activity does not exacerbate the pain. Still, his doctor gave him some triptan samples to try. Much to their surprise, the triptans worked. With no family history of Migraine and not trusting a diagnosis of Migraine, Randy's neurologist referred him to another neurologist with more experience in head trauma. The second neuro confirmed the diagnosis of post-traumatic headache. Randy's case demonstrates a couple of points about post-traumatic headache:*

▌ *They can begin years after the original trauma.*
▌ *Although we generally think triptans are effective only for Migraine attacks or cluster headaches, post-traumatic headaches are often Migraine-like and may respond to Migraine-specific treatments.*

Post-traumatic headaches can be among the most difficult to diagnose and treat. We rather expect to have a headache immediately following a head trauma, so a headache at that point doesn't surprise anyone. However, as shown in the second case example, not all post-traumatic headaches begin immediately following the trauma. Post-traumatic headaches can take many forms. Thus, there is no set treatment recommendation. It's important that the treating physician(s) listen to the patient, carefully evaluate the symptoms of the particular headache presentation, then choose appropriate treatment. As with other forms of head pain disorders, post-traumatic headaches can be classified as acute or chronic, depending on their frequency. In nature they can be similar to tension-type headache, the head pain of a Migraine attack, or other head pain. Selection of treatment depends on the character the headache takes on. As demonstrated in Randy's case, since his headaches had Migraine-like characteristics, Migraine-specific medications were the best choice for him. Patti did better with medications used for treating tension-type headaches.

When post-traumatic headaches are chronic, care must be taken not to exacerbate the situation by entering into an analgesic rebound situation. Working toward an effective preventive regimen is a wise choice in these cases. When you are choosing preventive medications, special considerations come into play:

- An injury and the resulting disruption to one's life can be very disturbing and create a situation perfect for the development of depression. In such circumstances, antidepressants that work well for headache prevention can sometimes do double duty.
- If the head trauma has caused any seizure activity, neuronal stabilizing agents (antiseizure medications) may be the best choice.
- In cases where back or neck injury accompanied the head injury, muscle relaxants, nerve blocks, physical therapy, and other therapies may be appropriate.

These are also cases in which it can be especially important for our medical teams to be willing to work together and to communicate with us. Be aware of that from the beginning. Once communication starts to slip, it can be quite difficult to get it back on track. This is also a time not to forget that the injury that started the headaches has also started changes in family dynamics. Children may feel frightened and insecure. Everyone will need reassurance. Don't be afraid to ask for help for your family if it's needed.

New Daily Persistent Headache

EXAMPLE CASE: *Tim had only had "regular" headaches on occasion—until he got one that just wouldn't go away, no matter what he did. The problem wasn't that the pain was severe. It wasn't. The pain was moderate, bilateral (on both sides), band-like, and movement didn't make it any worse. He was also experiencing some mild photophobia (sensitivity to light). His family doctor told him to take acetaminophen. Right. Since it didn't help, Tim took it for only a couple of days. Lucky Tim. He didn't know about analgesic rebound headache, but he saved himself from it. After a few months of what Tim refers to as "that nonsense," he insisted upon being referred to a neurologist. A CAT scan and MRI were negative. A lumbar puncture was negative. The neurologist was stumped and wrote Tim a prescription for Vicodin but did warn him about rebound headache. In the dark as to what he was supposed to do about a headache that never went away and medication that he was to take only a couple of days a week, Tim pushed his family doctor and insurance company for a referral to a headache specialist. That's where he first heard about new daily persistent headache. Since Tim experienced photophobia with his headache, the specialist theorized that triptans might be helpful in his treatment. He is currently alternating triptans and pain medications to avoid rebound issues while pursuing effective preventive medications.*

New daily persistent headache (NDPH) is headache that is daily and unremitting from very soon after it first occurs (within three days at most). The pain is generally on both sides, pressing or tightening in quality, and of mild to moderate intensity. There may be mild nausea, phonophobia (sensitivity to sound), or photophobia (sensitivity to light). Headache may be unremitting from the time it begins, or it may very rapidly build up to continuous and unremitting pain. Such onset or rapid development must be clearly recalled and unqualifiedly described by the patient to be diagnosed as NDPH. The headache must also meet these IHS criteria:

▌ Headache for more than three months fulfilling the following:
  * *Headache is daily and unremitting from onset or from less than three days from onset*
  * *Pain has at least two of the following characteristics:*

- bilateral (on both sides) location
- pressing/tightening quality (not pulsating)
- mild or moderate in intensity
- not aggravated by routine physical activity such as walking or climbing stairs
- *Both of the following:*
  - no more than one of mild nausea, phonophobia (sensitivity to sound), or photophobia (sensitivity to light)
  - neither moderate or severe nausea nor vomiting

As you look at those symptoms, you may notice that they resemble those of the tension-type headache in some respects and Migraine disease in others. The pain has the characteristics of TTH, but the nausea, phonophobia (sensitivity to sound), or photophobia (sensitivity to light) are characteristic of Migraine attacks, not TTH. As you think about that, can you take a guess as to how NDPH might be treated? Hint: Think about post-traumatic headache treatment. Right. NDPH is also treated according to the symptoms it presents in each individual patient. If it most resembles TTH, TTH-appropriate treatments are tried first. If it most resembles Migraine, Migraine-appropriate treatments are tried. The final treatment regimen may well be a combination, both in acute medications and in preventives. NDPH is still very much a mystery. There is some indication that it may be postviral in some patients, but there isn't enough evidence to support this as a main theory. Prognosis is a mystery. Sometimes NDPH stops as suddenly and mysteriously as it began.

Summary

Obviously we can't cover every type of head pain disorder here, but we've covered those that any of us are most likely to encounter.

Even as this book goes to press, journal articles are coming out with new information. It may sound strange, but it's almost an exciting time to be living with a headache disorder because of the progress being made. There's more information available than ever before, better medications, more research being conducted. Onward!

PART TWO

Your Health Care Team and Treatment Regimen

9

Your Role on Your Health Care Team

Optimal health care can be achieved only when patients are educated about their health and patients and physicians work together as treatment partners in an atmosphere of mutual respect.

It's critical that *we* be active members of our health care teams. Those of us with chronic headaches and Migraine disease need to be able to make basic treatment decisions when we have a headache or Migraine. We need to decide what medication to take and when to take it. It's just not possible to call our doctors each time. Especially with Migraine, if we educate ourselves about the whole disease, we can often notice signs of an impending attack and be prepared to take medication early enough to avoid a full-blown, debilitating episode.

We're actually fortunate to be living when we are. There is more information available today than ever before, partly because of the Internet. Where I live, the library doesn't have medical journals, and books on medical topics tend to be few and hardly new. The bookstores here don't have many choices either. That made my sources of information very limited until I got Internet access. Of course, when you surf the Internet for information, you do have to be particular about the sites you trust. That takes a while to figure out, but it's worth it. We now have instant access to governmental sites such as the National Institutes of Health, sites of nonprofit organizations founded for patient education and advocacy, sites to access medical journals, and other excellent sites brimming with helpful information. We also have the wonderful online bookstores where we can find just about any book we might desire.

Don't let anyone fool you. *Knowledge is power, and lack of knowledge is one reason people have felt so powerless against their health issues in the past.* Even people in my parents' generation would never have thought to ask their doctors questions. They went to the doctor, then did or didn't do what the doctor said to do. They took their medications without thinking to ask about possible side effects. They didn't ask what they could do for themselves to improve their condition. Most of all, it would have taken a great deal for them to ever doubt a doctor. The first time I fired a doctor for telling me my Migraines were a "female thing" I'd have to live with, my mother was shocked. What did I think I was doing? He was a doctor, so he knew what he was talking about; what did I know about medicine?

We are changing, and the practice of medicine is slowly changing. More and more, we ask those questions, will go to another doctor if we don't feel our treatment is correct and adequate, and are beginning to realize that we are ultimately responsible for our own health.

So who should be in charge of our health care team? Answer these questions:

- Who is with our bodies 24/7?
- Who knows our symptoms best?

- ■ Who is most impacted by how we feel?
- ■ Who is most affected by the success or failure of our treatment?
- ■ Who pays the $$ for the appointment or for the insurance that pays for the appointment?
- ■ Who is ultimately responsible for our lives and our health?

The answer? We are? Right! Therefore, we should be in charge of our health care team. We need to find doctors who are willing to work with us as treatment partners. That means that they give us the same respect they expect from us. That means they listen to us, don't mind answering questions, and don't resent that we are educated "consumers" in the health care market. When doctors work with us as treatment partners, they don't make decisions for us, they make decisions with us. Doctors who work this way say it's much more effective. When patients take part in the decision-making process, they're more compliant patients and stick to treatment plans far better.

How an Effective Health Care Team Should Work

So far, we've determined that we're ultimately responsible for our health and that we should be in charge of our health care team. Our partner in this should be our primary care physician, family doctor, internist, whoever is your primary doctor. I'll just refer to that doctor as our PCP. Our PCP sees to as many of our medical needs as possible, referring us to specialists as needed.

We should be able to expect any specialists we need to see to work with us in the same fashion we expect our PCPs to work with us: as treatment partners. Those specialists should automatically be sending regular reports to our PCP and should be willing to send reports to other doctors at our request. If any aspect of treatment with a specialist has the potential to affect a health issue being treated by another specialist or our PCP, it is quite reasonable to ask that specialist to consult with the other specialist or our PCP. It is not our job as patients to be go-betweens. Each person who is added to the communication chain between doctors increases the chances of miscommunication or confusion.

Where specialists are concerned, don't hesitate to let your PCP know if you have concerns about a specialist he or she sends you to. He needs to know if there are problems, and if it's just a misunderstanding, he may be able to resolve the issue. If necessary, he can refer you to a different specialist.

Doing Our Part

Many things go into doing our part to be an effective part of our health care team:

▮ *Keep learning:* This can't be emphasized too much. Learn about good health, good nutrition, and any conditions you have. The return on your investment here will be astonishing.

▮ *Talk about medications:* Doctors are human. To be on the safe side, when given a prescription for a new medication, ask if new medications are safe with any other medications you're taking. Don't forget to mention any over-the-counter medications, herbal medications, and dietary supplements you may be taking. Also ask what effect you can expect to see from the medication and what potential side effects to watch for. When you pick up your prescription at the pharmacy, read the patient information sheet carefully before you leave the pharmacy. That gives you a chance to ask the pharmacist any questions you may have at that time.

▌ *Provide information:* Keep your headache or Migraine diary current as well as any other notes on symptoms or events that you need to tell your doctor about at your next appointment. If you do this on the computer or transfer it to the computer, you can print two copies for your appointment—one for the doctor and one for yourself. That way, you can both be looking at it as you discuss it.

▌ *Be organized:* As you think of questions you want to ask at your next appointment, write them down or start a document on your computer. Before your appointment, get them typed up on the computer. Leave space between them so you can take notes. Again, make two copies so you and the doctor can look at them as you discuss them. Similarly, if you take several medications, it's helpful to keep a list on your computer of your medications, the dosages, and instructions. Take a copy with you whenever you go to the doctor to save the nurse time when he or she's checking to see what has changed from your last appointment. This list also comes in handy when you need to see a specialist or even when you go to the dentist. For your doctor, you can also make a note of how many to dispense and how many refills for the purpose of writing new prescriptions for you. They and their nurses have so many different patients and insurance plans to keep up with that it's very helpful to them when you can hand them a list of exactly what you need and how you need it written. It also saves you the time it can take to have to get a new prescription if one is written wrong or the trouble of straightening things out if one is written wrong and you fill it without noticing.

▌ *Be patient about waiting:* We all hate it when we're kept sitting in the waiting room or in the exam room. However, to me, if the doctor takes his time with me when he or she comes in, that does a lot to mitigate the waiting. For many reasons, doctors now have to fit quite a few patients into a day's schedule. Some also work emergencies into each day's routine. I know there have been times with some of my doctors that they've spent more than the allotted time with me, putting them behind for their next patient. So as long as the doctor takes the appropriate amount of time with me and doesn't rush through the appointment, I'm now just resigned to some waiting time.

▌ *Accept nurse practitioners and physician's assistants:* There may be times when you don't feel well and your doctor's schedule is packed. At such times, you may be scheduled to see his nurse practitioner or physician's assistant. Realize that they are well-trained medical professionals in their own right and give them a chance. They, too, can be valuable members of your health care team. You may even discover that for some appointments you'd prefer to see them instead of the doctor.

▌ *Remember to say, "Thank you":* Anyone who deals with the public gets a lot of complaints but few compliments and little thanks. When you consider that doctors and their staff are dealing with people who are ill a great deal of the time, that has to make it even more stressful. It will work in your favor to be one of the few who sincerely thank them and compliment them for their caring attitude and helpfulness. It's easy to forget to thank people when you're ill or even just focused on health issues, but it's the right thing to do and well worth the effort.

▌ *Follow our regimen, evaluate, and report:* Between appointments, it's our job to follow the treatment regimen we've agreed upon, note progress or minor problems that don't necessitate a call to the doctor, and report back at the next appointment so necessary changes can be made.

■ *Don't accept less than you deserve:* Although this is the last item listed here, it's not the least important. I left it for last to set it apart because it is vitally important. I know all too well how easy it is to stay with a doctor and just coast along because it's simpler than making the decision to move on. That said, we deserve better than that. We deserve the best health care team possible, and if we and our doctors aren't working well together as treatment partners, for whatever reason, and it can't be remedied, then we do ourselves a disservice if we accept less. Sometimes the doctor and/or the staff are really nice people, and we don't want to hurt their feelings, but we're not making progress. There are also situations where we may not be all that thrilled with the doctor, but even the thought of looking for a new doctor and starting over is exhausting and somewhat overwhelming. Oh, yes. Most of us have been there, haven't we? Stop and give it serious consideration, though. If we're not making progress, communication isn't good, or our headaches or Migraines are getting even worse, "doing our part" includes replacing part of our health care team. In some instances, it doesn't have to be difficult. Often, doctors will realize that a case isn't progressing and suggest referring us to another doctor. If they haven't done that yet, but we've been working with them for a reasonable length of time without results, some doctors are relieved if we bring up the subject and ask if they think it's time for another opinion. Regardless, it's a good idea to periodically ask our doctor how he or she thinks our case is progressing.

That gives you an opening to express your concern if no progress is being made. If it comes down to having to make the decision to move on to another doctor, we're only looking out for our health and well-being. Ultimately, that's our responsibility.

10

Choosing the Right Doctor

The logical place to start is with our family physician. He or she is the doctor who knows us best and can usually diagnose head pain. If your family doctor can't give you an accurate diagnosis or doesn't know how to treat you, a neurologist should be your next step. Keep in mind that neurologists aren't necessarily headache and Migraine specialists, but they should be better able to help you than your family physician. Many headache and Migraine patients do very well under the care of a neurologist.

General practice neurologists see patients with many conditions and injuries. That makes it virtually impossible for them to have extensive experience in any one particular area or to stay totally up-to-date in any one particular area. If you see a neurologist who says he or she can't help you or you haven't made progress after being treated for a reasonable period of time, it's time to move on to a headache and Migraine specialist. Unfortunately, it's important to note that it takes very little for some doctors to call themselves "specialists." Thus, I recommend that you seek care from a reputable specialist with an established track record. I keep a directory of recommended specialists that I compile based on patient recommendations. You can access that directory at www.HelpForHeadaches. com/lwfiles/specialists.htm. The American Council for Headache Education has a "Physician Finder" at www.achenet.org/physicians, and MAGNUM, the National Migraine Association, has a directory at www.migraines.org/help/helpclin.htm.

In some cases, our family physicians are the only doctors we need to see. In other cases, a neurologist, headache and Migraine specialist, ophthalmologist, endocrinologist, cardiologist, or other doctor may need to be consulted or even become an ongoing part of our medical team. It's essential that all our doctors be willing to consult one another and work together. No illness or condition exists totally independently. They all affect our overall health, and sooner or later, it's usually necessary for doctors to communicate to avoid treatment conflicts. If your doctors aren't willing to work that way, fire their sorry butts and find real doctors who will. We deserve no less.

How *Do* You Choose the Right Doctor?

Choosing the right doctor is a combination of doing our homework before making an appointment, then asking the right questions once we get there.

Doing Our Homework

▪ If you are choosing a specialist, get recommendations from your primary doctor. Don't hesitate to ask just how much your doctor actually knows about the specialist. You can also ask your doctor if he or she can arrange for you to talk to another patient who has been referred to the specialist.

▪ Remember that your pharmacist is a member of your health

care team and often a good source of information. Pharmacists frequently know quite a bit about doctors.

▮ Talk to the nurses at your doctor's office and any nurses who may be friends. Nurses also tend to know quite a bit about doctors.

▮ Talk with friends, especially any who also have headaches or Migraine disease. See what they know about the doctor you're considering. Ask who their doctors are, how they are to work with, and so on. The best indicator is generally firsthand feedback from another patient.

Asking the Right Questions

It's probably important to note for this section that I've had some great experiences with doctors and some pretty rotten experiences as well. There were times when I stayed with less than great doctors, but those times are over. I have now "fired" a few doctors, too. Don't get me wrong. I respect doctors, but I expect them to both deserve my respect and to return it. So the first few questions in this section are about how the doctor works with his or her patients and what you want and can expect from the doctor. Not everyone will be comfortable with these questions, so you can, of course, just not use them. They are here because they are questions I always want answered before I decide if I am even going to begin treatment with a particular doctor.

Questions About the Doctor and His or Her Practice

I'll suggest the questions here, but you'll want to phrase them in a way that's natural for you.

▮ I want to be an active part of my health care team. How do you feel about the team approach, with the patient and doctor working together as treatment partners?

- ▌ Not because I question your judgment, but because I want to understand and learn, I tend to ask quite a few questions. Will this bother you?
- ▌ Will you be the doctor I see every time I have an appointment here? (This is for group practices.)
- ▌ What's the procedure if I need assistance outside of office hours?

Questions About Headache and Migraine Treatment

- ▌ What is the diagnosis for my head pain? (tension-type headache, Migraine disease, and so forth)
- ▌ Exactly what is happening in my body during these episodes?
- ▌ Are there lifestyle changes I can make to help prevent these headaches and/or Migraines?
- ▌ What might be triggering these headaches and/or Migraines?
- ▌ Are the episodes frequent enough to consider preventive medications?
- ▌ Regarding medications being prescribed:
  - What type of drug is this, and how does it work?
  - If prescribing more than one drug, what should be taken when, and in what order?
  - What are the possible side effects? Will they go away? At what point should I call you about any side effects?
  - What is this drug's potential to cause rebound headache? If I've already used it as many consecutive days as it can safely be used without risking rebound, what can I take instead?
- ▌ If nausea is a problem, and the doctor does not offer to prescribe an antinausea drug, it would be a good idea to ask for one. (Reglan, Phenergan, Compazine, and so forth)
- ▌ If there has been a significant change in headache patterns,

and your doctor is not ordering an imaging study (CAT scan or MRI), ask if the doctor thinks it would be advisable.

▪ If you awaken feeling unrested, experience excessive daytime sleepiness, or already know you have sleep problems, be sure to discuss this with your doctor. Sleep patterns are essential to your health and to preventing headaches and Migraines.

▪ Does the doctor suggest any vitamin or mineral supplements—magnesium, vitamin B_2, coenzyme Q_{10}, or others? If so, what and in what amount?

▪ Does the doctor suggest herbal remedies such as feverfew? Again, in what amounts?

There are many other questions you may want to ask that will pertain to your individual situation, but this is a beginning. To make things a bit easier for you, I've made these questions available online at HelpForHeadaches.com/lwfiles/new-doc-questions.htm. You can print the page, copy and paste the questions into your word processor, or customize them to your use.

Two Notes About Specialists

▪ Neurologists are not necessarily headache and Migraine specialists. They treat a wide range of neurological illnesses and diseases as well as injuries involving neurological problems. There are headache and Migraine specialists who treat nothing else. That means they have far more experience in the field. They also have more time to devote to staying up-to-date on diagnosis and treatment.

▪ For the most part, doctors who call themselves specialists are specialists. Unfortunately, I've talked to too many people who went to a doctor who was supposed to be a headache and Migraine specialist, only to discover that this particular "specialist" didn't know any more than their family doctor and was unable to help them. This is why I recommend checking out a specialist before making an appointment.

The Pep Talk

Even though I'm going to be repeating myself, a pep talk is appropriate here. Years of working with headache sufferers and Migraineurs who have had good and bad experiences with their doctors, as well as personal experience, have shown me just how difficult it can be to change doctors. We get frustrated, even angry, but then back down and keep going back to the same doctor. Does that sound familiar? I thought so. If you're one of my online readers, you know what's coming. Our doctors work for us. Period. They don't pay us to go to those appointments. If we're not making progress, they don't take enough time with us, they don't answer questions, or they don't give us as much respect as they expect to receive, it's time to fire their sorry butts and move on! Every day we delay is one day longer we spend in pain without making progress. If you're in that situation, repeat after me: "I *will* fire his [or her] sorry butt!" Okay? Okay!

11

Trigger Identification and Management

Before discussing triggers, we need to clarify that "cause" and "trigger" are not the same thing. Too often the terms are used interchangeably, leading to confusion. In previous chapters, we talked about cluster headaches being caused by activation of the hypothalamus and trigeminal nerve and Migraine disease being caused by overly excitable neurons (nerve cells that have the ability to transmit and receive nervous impulses) in our brains. Those are causes. Triggers are stimuli that in interaction with the body constitute a physiological trigger that brings on a headache or Migraine attack.

Tension-Type Headache Triggers

- stress
- missing meals
- cigarette smoke
- lack of sleep
- bright lights

Migraine Triggers

▌ certain foods: The best way to determine if you have food
triggers is by following an elimination diet where you cut
out all the potential trigger foods, then add them back into
your diet one at a time to see if any of them trigger a Migraine. The list of potential food triggers, when detailed, is
quite long (you can find a complete list of potential trigger
foods in many books or online at www.HelpForHeadaches.
com/lwfiles/trigger-foods.htm):

aged meats

alcoholic beverages, especially
red wines

apricots

artificial sweeteners

avocados

bacon

bananas

beans: navy, lima, pinto, string,
garbanzo, pole, lentils, snow
peas, fava, Italian

bologna

buttermilk

canned meats

canned soups (contain
monosodium glutamate)

capers

caviar

chili peppers

chocolate milk

citrus fruits

coconut

concentrated sugars

cream

cured meats

dates

figs

fresh yeast breads straight from
the oven, including breads,
crackers, doughnuts, pizza
dough, and soft pretzels

fresh yeast products

ham

hot dogs

ketchup

liver and other organ meats

mayonnaise

monosodium glutamate (MSG)

most cheeses

mustards

nuts

olive oil

olives

papayas

passion fruit

peanuts and peanut butter

pepperoni

pickles

processed meats

raisins

red plums

salami

sausage

seeds

soy sauce

sulfites

vinegar except cider and white
      vinegars

whole milk

- changes in weather
- disrupted, poor-quality, too much, or too little sleep
- fragrances such as perfumes or colognes
- fumes from cleaning products, pesticides, and paint
- dehydration
- missing meals
- hormone fluctuations
- fluorescent lighting
- flickering light such as strobe lights, flashing banner ads on Web pages, or even sunlight coming through trees as you travel along a road
- very bright lighting or very bright sunlight
- the nearly imperceptible flicker of some monitors, related to the refresh rate
- light glare
- crying
- crowded, stuffy rooms
- overly loud places
- high altitude
- idiopathic intracranial hypertension (IIH), aka pseudotumor cerebri: This is a bit off the beaten path and not especially common, but it can be worth checking out in some cases. With IIH, for no reason anyone has been able to discover, the body produces too much cerebrospinal fluid

(CSF), which makes the CSF pressure too high. Some patients with IIH present the symptom of papilledema (edema and inflammation of the optic nerve where it enters the retina) in an ophthalmic exam, but papilledema isn't always present. The definitive diagnostic test for IIH is a lumbar puncture (spinal tap) to measure the CSF pressure. With a gauge on the needle being used, measuring fluid is easy, and the pressure is known immediately. If it's beyond the normal range, fluid may be drawn off at that time to put the pressure into normal range. Usually, no other action is taken for a few weeks. This gives the doctor and patient the opportunity to see if there's a change in the Migraine pattern. If a reduction is seen, it's usually indicative that the pressure was indeed too high for the individual, and the pressure can usually be kept within the normal range with oral medications. When I started working with my Migraine specialist, I could identify my triggers only about 50 percent of the time. I usually had tinnitus (ringing, hissing, or buzzing sound in the ears) with those Migraines where I couldn't identify the trigger, and preventives just weren't working. He suggested a lumbar puncture to rule out IIH. It turned out that my CSF pressure was higher than the normal range, so he drew off fluid during the procedure. Three weeks later, I was able to report nearly a 50 percent reduction in the number of Migraine attacks and no tinnitus with my Migraines. It wasn't long before my preventives started showing promise.

Migraine triggers can be cumulative, or what Dr. Jan Brandes calls "stackable." In other words, there may well be times when you can encounter one or even more of your triggers without having a Migraine attack. Yet when one more trigger is added, a Migraine attack occurs. This is also sometimes referred to as your "trigger threshold." Some triggers may be stronger for you than others and can trigger a Migraine by themselves.

One thing I'd like to point out is that stress itself is not a Migraine trigger. It's what's termed an exacerbating factor. It doesn't trigger Migraines, but it does make us more susceptible to our triggers. An analogy is the best way I know to explain it. When we're stressed, we're more likely to "catch a cold." It's not stress that causes the cold; it's the cold virus. The stress just made us more susceptible to the virus. Stress and Migraine have the same kind of relationship. Stress doesn't actually trigger a Migraine, but it makes us more susceptible to our triggers.

Cluster Headache Triggers

A cluster series tends to start on its own, without triggers. Once it starts, the individual headaches don't necessarily need triggers, but there are some things that can trigger them in some individuals:

- alcoholic beverages
- cigarette smoke
- monosodium glutamate (MSG)
- aged meats
- letdown after stress
- excessive cold or heat
- bright light

Identifying Triggers

Identifying triggers is easy for some people, not so easy for others. This is another time your headache and Migraine diary is valuable. While you're in the process of identifying triggers, you may want to supplement your diary with some kind of appointment journal so you can record places you go, the weather, what you ate, and other things that can give you clues.

Food triggers can be very difficult to identify. Often, the best way to identify them is through an elimination diet. In an elimination diet, you cut out all potential trigger foods, then add them back in, one at a time, to identify any triggers. Monosodium glutamate (MSG) is a fairly common Migraine trigger found in foods. Unfortunately, it's in many prepared and prepackaged foods and used in many restaurants. Another problem with MSG is that it's not always called MSG. Some other sources of MSG are autolyzed yeast, calcium caseinate, gelatin, hydrolyzed protein, sodium caseinate, and yeast extract.

Remember what Dr. Brandes said about triggers being "stackable"? That's something that can make identifying triggers difficult, too. Many of us have triggers that aren't strong enough to precipitate a headache or Migraine on their own but are when they're combined with another trigger. Thus, something that seems to be a trigger in one incident may not seem to be at another time.

Trigger Management

Obviously, there are some triggers over which we have no control, such as changes in the weather. However, those of us who do have triggers we can control have an advantage. That means there's something we can do for ourselves to prevent some of our headaches and Migraines. It tends to be busy in doctors' offices, so most of the time we're told to do what we can to avoid our triggers and that's it. I think it bears more discussion than that.

Make a list of your triggers in two columns—those you can avoid or control and those you can't. Discuss the list with your doctor for his or her suggestions. You might also want to discuss it with family, a friend, or a fellow headache or Migraine sufferer. They might think of some trigger avoidance methods that hadn't occurred to you. Let's also take a look at those triggers here:

- *Alcoholic beverages:* When a cluster headache sufferer is in the midst of a cluster cycle, just about anything alcoholic is a trigger if alcohol is a previously identified trigger. For Migraineurs, it can be a bit different. Red wine seems to be especially problematic because of the tyramine in it. Beer can be a problem because of the yeast. Some Migraineurs find they can drink white wine and some other alcoholic beverages without triggering a Migraine. Again, it's a process of elimination.
- *Stress:* Stress can trigger tension-type headaches and is an exacerbating factor in Migraines. It's also detrimental to our health. Thus, stress reduction is good for everyone. A certain amount of stress is good; it helps us perform better and be alert and productive. This good stress is called "eustress." Negative stress is called "distress." There are a number of ways to deal with distress. If there are stressful situations that can be resolved, that's a good place to start. We also have to learn to let go of stressors we can't change and cope better even with those we can change. Stress management expert Dr. Melissa C. Stöppler advises, "Develop your relaxation skills. Stress control requires your being able to put aside the demands and stressors in your daily life, at least temporarily. Many people have actually lost the ability to relax and create emotional distance from troubling thoughts and may need to retrain their body and mind to relax effectively." Personally, two things have enabled me to achieve healthy stress management:
  - *Each morning, I start out by taking thirty minutes of absolute "me time." Depending on how I feel, I either sit on*

> *a pillow on my office floor or at the table. I light a mildly scented candle and close the curtains. Then I spend thirty minutes praying, meditating, and getting myself centered and focused for the day ahead.*

- *Whether I'm feeling stressed or not, I also take time to listen to my favorite relaxation CD at some point during the late afternoon or evening. This advice was given to me by my Migraine specialist after my Migraines had been brought under fairly good control, as an aid to maintaining overall good health. You don't have a favorite relaxation CD? You can try mine! It's* Effortless Relaxation *by Steven Halpern. You can check it out on his Web site, www. stevenhalpern.com, or in many stores.*

▌ *Cigarette smoke:* This one makes some people unhappy. The bottom line here is that we sometimes have to make a lifestyle choice and give up going to clubs and parties where there will be a lot of cigarette smoke. At private parties, it seems to be less of a problem than in the past, because fewer people are smoking and more homes are smoke-free. When you are invited to a private party, it's perfectly acceptable to ask the host or hostess in advance if people will be smoking. If it's an outdoors party, that makes things much easier.

▌ *Disrupted, poor-quality, too much, or too little sleep:* For some people, this is going to be a trigger over which you have quite a bit of control; for others, not. Parents with infants and small children will find this a problem until their children are sleeping peacefully through the night. This one is also problematic for shift workers. You just get settled into a sleep rhythm, then you change shifts. If staying on one shift is a possibility, and sleep is a trigger for you, discuss this with your supervisor. For those who can do it, the best solution is to set a regular time to go to bed each night and get up each morning. If you don't sleep well or get up feeling as tired as when you went to bed, talk to your doctor about a sleep study. I can attest to this one firsthand. I thought I was sleeping well, but I was waking with Migraines. After asking several questions, my doctor sent me for a sleep study. It turned out that I had two sleep disorders that were keeping me from getting enough REM-stage sleep. Once those were treated, I stopped waking up with Migraines so frequently.

■ *Fragrances such as perfumes or colognes:* This one is a mixed bag. You can do only so much about the people around you. If fragrance is a serious trigger for you at work, try talking with your co-workers. If that doesn't work, try talking to your supervisor. There will be more information on this in chapter 17. For yourself and your family, determine if it's all fragrances or just certain fragrances, perhaps heavy fragrances, and work from there. If it's all fragrances, look carefully at the ingredients on cosmetics, skin care products, and hair care products. Even if they're not perfumed, many of them have fragrance in them just to make them smell more pleasant. If all fragrances are triggers for you, and visitors to your home insist on wearing fragrance when they visit, you can always consider installing a fire hose outside your front door and keeping a supply of towels and bathrobes handy. Chances are they'll get the not-so-subtle hint after the first time!

■ *Fumes from cleaning products, pesticides, and paint:* This is another one that can go in both columns of your list. You can pretty much control these things at home, but not other places. At home, you may need to make arrangements to be away from home when painting is being done and pesticides are being used. As for cleaning products, there are "natural" products available, and you can make some cleaning products yourself from common kitchen items. Both baking soda and vinegar have many cleaning uses.

■ *Dehydration:* Here's one we can do a great deal to prevent. Repeat after me: "Water is my friend." It's true! Caffeinated drinks don't help with hydration, so don't count on them. Water is best. If you truly don't like drinking water, try it again with lots of ice, or try some of the flavored waters. I take a water bottle with me everywhere I go, even places that are posted "No Food or Drink." When someone says something to me, I point out that the bottle is sealed and that I need to carry water to prevent getting ill from dehydration.

■ *Missing meals:* There will be times when meals are late. That's life. If that tends to be a trigger for you, carry a snack with you that you can eat at the time you'd normally be eating your meal. Then get back on schedule as soon as possible. Sugary snacks are not the best choice for this purpose. Snacks with protein will do much better.

■ *Fluorescent lighting:* At home, you can pretty much control this. When you go shopping, take sunglasses and a sun visor or cap with a visor. The sunglasses should keep the fluorescent lighting from hitting the main part of your visual field. The visor will block the light that would come in over the top of the glasses. For many people, this is sufficient to allow them time in places with fluorescent lighting. Fluorescent lighting at work is another matter. Sunglasses and a visor can help but aren't very practical day in and day out for the full workday. How are the fluorescent tubes arranged in your workplace? Many people have solved this problem by explaining the situation and asking that the fluorescent tube(s) over their work space be removed. One person told me her company wouldn't allow the fixture to be empty, but when tubes burned-out in another area, they put the burned out tubes in the fixture over her work area. If the lighting fixtures aren't conducive to this solution, talk to your supervisor about moving you to a different work space where the problem can be addressed.

▌ *Very bright light, bright sunlight:* When you have to be outside on sunny days, shade is an obviously desirable thing. Even in the shade or on cloudy days, the sun and glare can be problematic. Migraineurs may even find that over time they become more sensitive to light in general, not just when they have Migraines. Invest in a pair of high-quality sunglasses; they can be very helpful both inside and outdoors. According to ophthalmologist Dr. Scott Strickler, there are some key points to observe:

• *Invest in good, optical-grade lenses that won't distort your vision or cause other problems.*

• *It's essential that the lenses be coated for both UVA and UVB rays. If not, the dark tint will make your exposure to UV rays worse by allowing your pupils to dilate and enabling more UV rays to enter the eye. UV rays have a cumulative effect on the eyes over the years and can contribute to later problems, including cataracts and macular degeneration.*

• *Polarized lenses are helpful because they reduce scattered light, which is what causes glare.*

As you look over the list of potential triggers, you may notice things such as dehydration, missed meals, or disrupted sleep. Do you see a commonality there? They're all things that are harmful to good overall health. When we're as healthy as possible, our bodies are less stressed, thus at their best to resist Migraine triggers. I know it's hard to think about a healthy lifestyle when you're plagued by chronic headaches or Migraine disease, but that healthy lifestyle can help reduce some triggers. Here are some goals:

▌ Drink enough water. If you're substituting other beverages for water, watch the caffeine; it can lead to dehydration.

▌ Eat well-balanced meals on a regular schedule.

▌ Go to bed at the same time each night and get up at the same time each morning, even on weekends and holidays.

▌ Work some exercise into your routine. I fully realize how difficult it is to exercise if you have a headache or Migraine, but do what you can. Here are some ways you can "sneak" some exercise into your days:

- *Park farther away from the door when you go shopping or run other errands. When you finish loading your groceries into your car, put the cart in the containment area in the parking lot. Those few extra steps add up.*

- *After you've been up a bit and aren't stiff, **remake your bed**. Stripping all the covers off your bed and remaking it is a great miniworkout with light lifting and stretching.*

- ***Work those stairs** at home. When you need to go up or down for something, turn around and do the stairs a second time. Away from home, whenever you have the choice of an elevator or stairs, take the stairs if you can. Even if you can't take the stairs going up, take them going down for a bit of exercise.*

- ***Pick up your feet.** If you're like me, you hated leg lifts in gym class, and they hurt your back now. It's not quite the same, but there is another way. Sit in a steady chair and lift one leg slowly until it's parallel with the floor. Hold for a few seconds, then lower it slowly. You can do this with your toe pointed away from you and with your toe pointed toward you to work different muscles. Then repeat with the other leg. As you get used to the activity, increase repetitions.*

- *Then **pick up some veggies**. Canned soup or vegetables are quite convenient to use as light hand weights. You can use* them to work on upper-body strength and/or range of motion. These exercises can be done one arm at a time, standing or sitting. Start with your arms straight at your side and bring them straight out to the side, pause level with the shoulder, then on up, straight toward the ceiling. Bring slowly back to your side. Do the same moving your arm forward. As you get used to these movements, increase the number of repetitions.

- **Dance with your Swiffer!** Nobody hates to dust the furniture and wipe down the walls, corner, and ceilings for cobwebs more than I do. So I pick a day when I feel pretty well, put on my favorite music, and dance away that dust! Don't be tempted to skip the top shelves or far corners. Again, stretching is good. If you're concerned about the neighbors wondering what you're doing, pull the draperies. Or don't—it's more fun to leave them wondering!

- **Stretch your wonderful self!** Careful, gentle stretching feels so good, and it's good for us. Stand with your feet shoulder-width apart. Slowly bring one arm up over your head and bend at the waist in the opposite direction. Repeat in the other direction. Gently bend forward at the waist as far as you can comfortably bend. If your balance is good, put one foot on a chair and bend your knee to stretch in. These may be done holding a chair if balance is a problem. You can also do lots of stretches sitting. If your balance is good, stretching in a hot shower is great!

- **Summon your inner child and play!** Take some time to play with your children, grandchildren, or pets. It's fun, lifts your spirits, and gives you a bit of exercise to boot!

12

Preventive Therapies

Preventive medications are taken daily to prevent headaches and Migraine attacks. It's almost impossible to express how important preventive therapies are and the wonderful changes they can bring to our lives. Most forms of head pain disorders respond to preventive therapies. While nobody wants to take medications on a daily basis, there are times when those daily medications can make such a vast improvement in one's health and life that the positives obviously outweigh the negatives. In the case of Migraine disease, there's another issue to remember. Migraineurs have a neurological disease. If we had another disease—say, thyroid disease or diabetes—we probably wouldn't hesitate to take the daily medications prescribed for us. We need to get our minds around the fact that Migraine, too, is a disease and adopt the same kind of attitude toward it.

Preventive therapies generally do more than reduce the frequency of headaches and Migraine attacks. They also usually reduce the severity of those that still occur, making them easier to treat and less debilitating. How's that for encouraging? My personal experience is that an effective preventive regimen allowed me to take one dose of a Migraine abortive medication and lose perhaps an hour or two at

Here's some good news: With all the medications and dietary supplements available today to be used as preventive therapies, plus the nearly endless combinations of them, effective preventive regimens can be found for at least 98 percent of headache and Migraine sufferers!

most out of my day rather than an entire day or two to a Migraine attack. My preventive regimen has essentially returned control of my life to *me*.

Migraine prevention is a perfect example of how medications that are developed for one condition often end up being very beneficial as treatments for other conditions. Several classes of medications originally intended to treat hypertension and/or heart disease are excellent Migraine preventives. Examples are beta blockers and calcium channel blockers. Several types of antidepressants have turned out to be quite helpful as Migraine preventives. Neuronal stabilizing agents, better known as antiseizure medications, are also being used for Migraine prevention. Although scientists haven't established what form it takes, they have strong theories that Migraine disease and epilepsy are related. That's one reason the neuronal stabilizing agents are so frequently prescribed for Migraine prevention.

The first of these antiseizure medications to be approved for Migraine prevention was Depakote. As I write this book, the only medications actually approved by the U.S. Food and Drug Administration (FDA) for Migraine prevention are Depakote (antiseizure medication), Inderal (beta-blocker), Blocadren (beta-blocker), and Topamax (antiseizure medication). Approximately one hundred other medications are being successfully prescribed off-label for Migraine prevention. Once approved by the FDA for one condition, doctors may prescribe medications off-label for other conditions if they have reason to believe they will be effective. Quite often this begins when patients who are taking a medication for one condition notice that it also helps with another one. That leads to small studies to test the efficacy of the medication for the second condition, then possibly to clinical trials. Off-label prescribing is quite common and has led to medications being found to be effective for other conditions far earlier than they might otherwise have been. This does sometimes present problems with insurance coverage of medications for off-label purposes, but this occurs in a relatively small percentage of cases.

[
Preventive medication should be started at a low dose and increased slowly until it starts working, side effects develop, or a maximum dose is reached.
—Young and Silberstein
]

Here's a list of medications I've compiled. These are medications I know are being used successfully by someone for Migraine and headache prevention. Some are commonly used and fairly well-known as Migraine and headache preventives. Others aren't well-known, but I know people for whom they work.

Antihypertensives (Blood Pressure Meds)

Alpha-2 Agonists
Clonidine, aka Catapres
Guanfacine, aka Tenex

ACE Inhibitors
Benazepril, aka Lotensin
Captopril, aka Capoten
Enalapril, aka Vasotec
Fosinopril, aka Monopril

Lisinopril, aka Zestril, Prinivil
Moexipril, aka Univasc
Perindopril, aka Aceon
Quinapril, aka Accupril
Ramipril, aka Altace
Trandolapril, aka Mavik

Angiotensin II Inhibitors
Candesartan, aka Atacand
Eprosartan, aka Teveten
Irbesartan, aka Avapro
Losartan, aka Cozaar
Olmesartan, aka Benicar
Telmisartan, aka Midcardis
Valsartan, aka Diovan

Beta Blockers
Acebutolol, aka Secral
Atenolol, aka Tenormin
Betaxolol, aka Kerlone
Bisoprolol, aka Zebeta, Emconcor
Cartelol, aka Cartrol
Labetalol, aka Normodyne, Trandate
Metoprolol, aka Lopressor, Toprol
Nadolol, aka Corgard
Penbutololm aka Levatol
Pindolol, aka Visken, Syn-Pindolol
Propranolol, aka Inderal
Timolol, aka Blocadren

Calcium Channel Blockers
Amlodipine, aka Norvasc
Bepridil, aka Vascor

Diltiazem, aka Cardizem, Tiazac
Felodipine, aka Plendil
Flunarizine, aka Sibelium (Canada)
Isradipine, aka DynaCirc
Nicardipine, aka Cardene
Nifedipine, aka Adalat, Procardia
Nimodipine, aka Nimotop
Nisoldipine, aka Sular
Verapamil, aka Calan, Verelan, Isoptin

Antihistamines

Cyproheptadine, aka Periactin
Pizotifen, aka Sandomigran (U.K.)

Antidepressants

Tricyclic Antidepressants (TCAs)

Amitriptyline, aka Elavil (brand-name Elavil no longer manufactured), Endep, Levate, Triptil
Amoxapine, aka Asendin
Clomipramine, aka, Anafranil
Desipramine, aka Norpramin
Doxepin, aka Sinequan
Imipramine, aka Norfranil, Tofranil
Nortriptyline, aka Pamelor, Aventyl
Protriptyline, aka Vivactil
Trimipramine, aka Surmontil

Monoamine Oxidase Inhibitor (MAOI) Antidepressants
Isocarboxazid, aka Marplan

Phenelzine, aka Nardil

Tranylcypromine, aka Parnate

Selective Serotonin Reuptake Inhibitors (SSRIs)
Citalopram, aka Celexa

Escitalopram oxalate, aka Lexapro

Fluoxetine, aka Prozac

Fluvoxamine, aka Luvox

Paroxetine, aka Paxil

Sertraline, aka Zoloft

Selective Serotonin and Norepinephrine Reuptake Inhibitors (SSNRIs)
Duloxetine, Cymbalta

Other Antidepressants
Bupropion, aka Wellbutrin, Zyban

Mirtazepine, aka Remeron

Trazodone, aka Desyrel

Venlafaxine, aka Effexor, Effexor XR

Arthritis Meds

Cox-2 Enzyme Inhibitors
Celecoxib, aka Celebrex

Note: Two other Cox-2 enzyme inhibitors, Bextra and Vioxx, were being prescribed prior to being removed from the market. Vioxx had also been approved by the FDA for pain relief during a Migraine attack.

Neuronal Stabilizing Agents (Antiseizure Meds)

Carbamazepine, aka Tegretol
Clonazepam, Klonopin
Clorazepate, aka Tranxene
Divalproex, aka Depakote
Gabapentin, aka Neurontin
Levetiracetam, Keppra
Lamotrigine, aka Lamictal
Oxcarbazepine, Trileptal
Tiagabine, aka Gabitril
Topiramate, aka Topamax
Valproate sodium, aka Depacon
Zonisamide, aka Zonegran

Ergot Alkaloid
Methylergonovine, aka Methergine (the only ergot used as a preventive)

Leukotriene Blockers
Montelukast, aka Singulair
Zafirlukast, aka Accolate
Zyleuton, aka Zyflo

Other
Baclofen, aka Lioresal
Botulinum toxin type A, aka Botox

Dietary Supplements
Coenzyme Q_{10}
Feverfew
Butterbur, aka Petadolex
Magnesium

Vitamin B$_2$

5-HTP (Check carefully with doctor because of interactions with
    meds, including triptans)

Lecithin

Melatonin

Combination supplements such as MigraLieve, MigraHealth, Mi-
    graVent, and so on

Botox is used as a preventive for headache and Migraine patients whose triggers involve certain muscles of the head and neck. The effects of Botox can last up to three or four months. The most common site for the injections is the forehead. Botox is a sterile, vacuum-dried form of purified botulinum toxin type A. Botox is to be reconstituted with sterile nonpreserved saline before injection.

A note of caution about Botox: As of spring 2005, only one company can legally sell Botox for human use, Allergan. At this time, several people are under arrest and being prosecuted for injecting people with "fake" Botox. This can be very dangerous—fatal, in fact. Be sure anyone injecting you with Botox is legitimate and using the genuine product!

Dietary Supplements as Preventives

On the list of preventive medications, you'll notice several vitamins, herbs, and minerals—dietary supplements. Like anything else, they don't work for everyone, and you'll know if they work for you only by trying them. However, please consult your doctor before trying any of them. These "natural" sources are precisely where society got our first drugs, and these substances act as drugs in our systems. If you already take a multivitamin or other supplements, you'll also need to check them to see if they contain any of these and, if so, in what amounts. You need to be sure you don't end up taking too much of something.

Preventive Therapies for Children and Adolescents

The American Academy of Neurology Quality Standards Subcommittee and the Practice Committee of the Child Neurology Society set out to review evidence on pharmacological treatment of children and adolescents with Migraine disease, analyze that evidence, and establish treatment guidelines. The team identified and studied 166 articles on pediatric treatment from peer-reviewed medical journals. Based on its review of all the available data, it made the following recommendations regarding Migraine prevention in children and adolescents:

1. Flunarizine is probably effective and could be considered but is not available in the United States.
2. There is insufficient evidence to make any recommendations concerning the use of cyproheptadine (Periactin), amitriptyline (Elavil), divalproex sodium (Depakote), topiramate (Topamax), or levetiracetam (Keppra).
3. Because the evidence is conflicting, recommendations cannot be made concerning propranolol (Inderal) or trazodone (Desyrel).
4. Pizotifen (Sandomigraine) and nimodipine (Nimotop) and clonidine did not show efficacy and are not recommended.

Dr. Donald W. Lewis, a pediatric head pain specialist affiliated with Children's Hospital of the King's Daughter in Norfolk, Virginia, was the lead author on the group's findings. During an interview, he commented:

This is one of those unfortunate areas where a very common problem has been understudied. There is a lot of denial, among families and among clinicians, that children do get Migraines. We need more clinical trials to see how these medicines work in children. . . . One of the themes here is that initial trials have failed. More intense and innovative research needs to be done.

Please read the findings carefully. Note that they do not say none of the medications mentioned work. They say there is insufficient or conflicting data and they cannot make recommendations about what works best. Anecdotally, I can tell you of parents who report to me that Inderal, Periactin, or Depakote have helped their children.

A Preventive Device

Not all preventives are medications or supplements. Most notably, a dental device called the NTI Tension Suppression System is now FDA-approved for chronic tension-type headache and Migraine prevention. It's a small device worn at night by people who tend to clench their teeth, thus strongly contracting the temporalis muscle. For some Migraineurs, this can be a trigger that often results in waking with Migraines as well as Migraines at other times of the day. It can also trigger tension-type headaches. James P. Boyd, D.D.S., inventor of the device, explains on his Web site:

When the temporalis contracts with extreme intensity during the normal REM sleep stage, the patient can be awakened from sleep with greater than usual head pain, or awakens in the morning with a greater than their "normal" degree of discomfort, which they then categorize as a headache.

Complete information about this device is available from Dr. Boyd's Web site, www.headacheprevention.com.

Summary

Beyond the obvious reasons for finding an effective preventive regimen, there are other considerations. The effects of chronic pain and other symptoms that can accompany headaches and Migraine attacks aren't exactly easy on our bodies. Days spent with headaches or Migraines reduce our activity and "normal" lifestyle. Many people find themselves gaining weight because of a reduction in physical activity. It's actually healthier for us to reduce the number of headaches and/or Migraine attacks we have.

It's only fair to tell you that it takes a while to know if a medication is going to work for prevention. Some medications need to be taken for up to three months before you give up on them. You'll notice that I never said finding effective preventives was easy. I just said it can be done for the vast majority of us, and that's true. It can definitely try one's patience, but once you've found the right regimen, you'll be ecstatic that you didn't give up. Just think of it this way— you have the strength and endurance to do this. Once you've found your regimen, you'll have all that strength and endurance to put into something you want to do!

Too many times, I've had people tell me that one preventive medication or another was producing a certain side effect. When I tell them that side effect is listed in the prescribing information for the medication, all too often they tell me that their doctor didn't mention it. Some doctors are quite thorough in telling you the potential side effects of medications they prescribe, some aren't. It's as if they think you're more likely to experience the side effects if they tell you they're a possibility. There may be a bit of validity in that. However, the far better approach is to know what effects could occur but assume they won't happen to you. Some of the medications used for headache and Migraine prevention are very serious drugs with possibly serious potential side effects. In a very few cases, there are medications that have potential side effects that can cause permanent damage, such as vision loss from glaucoma. Be wise about these and all medications. Ask your doctor about potential side effects. Be sure your pharmacist gives you an information sheet on all your prescriptions, and read them. If you have questions, ask your doctor or pharmacist. Report any side effects you experience to your doctor. Do not take chances. Preventive medications are wonderful, and they can help return control of our lives to us, but we have to treat them with caution and respect. Be safe.

13

Abortive Therapies

Abortive therapies are not painkiller medications. Pain medications mask pain for the period of time of their action. Abortive medications actually work at the source of a Migraine attack, cluster headache, or Migraine-like headache. They work to return neurotransmitter levels to normal, stop the attack completely, and relieve all the associated symptoms.

Today, the most commonly prescribed abortive medications are the triptans:

▌ Sumatriptan (Imitrex, Imigran): Introduced in the United States in 1992 in injectable form. Now also available in tablets and nasal spray.

▌ Zolmitriptan (Zomig): Introduced in the United States in tablet form in 1997. Orally dissolvable tablets introduced in 2001, nasal spray in 2003.

▌ Naratriptan (Amerge, Naramig): Introduced in the United States in tablet form in 1998.

▌ Rizatriptan (Maxalt): Introduced in the United States in

tablet form in 1998. Orally dissolvable tablets introduced later in 1998.

▌ Almotriptan (Axert): Introduced in the United States in tablet form in 2001.

▌ Frovatriptan (Frova): Introduced in the United States in tablet form in 2001.

▌ Eletriptan (Relpax): Introduced in the United States in tablet form in 2002.

The triptans are wonderful medications for those who can take them and those for whom they're effective. They're effective for approximately 80 percent of Migraineurs. For patients for whom the triptans are intended and prescribed correctly, their safety is proving remarkable. After reviewing dozens of studies and adverse event reports on triptans from the FDA's Adverse Event Reporting System, the Triptan Cardiovascular Safety Expert Panel of the American Headache Society (AHS) has come to a conclusion vital to those who suffer from Migraines and cluster headaches. Referring to patients who have no risks of cardiovascular disease, Dr. David Dodick commented, "While serious cardiovascular events have been reported after the use of triptans, their occurrence appears to be extremely low—on the order of less than 1 in 1 million." Such figures put triptans in a better safety position than over-the-counter nonsteroidal anti-inflammatory medications such as ibuprofen, acetaminophen, and aspirin. The risk of death from those medications is as little as 1 in 1,200, while prescription NSAIDs contribute to approximately 16,500 deaths per year.

Because their vasoconstrictive properties cannot be totally confined to the blood vessels affected by Migraine, they should not be take by people who have uncontrolled hypertension, a history of heart disease or stroke, or strong risk factors for either heart disease or stroke or by Migraineurs who experience hemiplegic or basilar-type Migraine.

Fallacy: Some people (unfortunately including a few doctors) think triptans work for all Migraineurs and that if triptans don't work, the patient can't have Migraine disease. This is *not* true. If a doctor says this to you—run! (Or laugh, but don't believe it!)

What Are Triptans and How Do They Work?

To understand triptans, we need to understand a few basic terms:

- *Neurotransmitters:* Chemicals occurring naturally in the brain that transmit messages from one nerve cell to another. In discussing Migraine, we talk most often about the neurotransmitter serotonin. Another involved in Migraine is norepinephrine.
- *Receptor:* A structure in the cell membrane that combines with a drug, hormone, infectious particle, or chemical to alter the function of the cell.
- *Agonist:* A drug that shows an affinity for and stimulates a receptor.
- *Selective* (in this context): Nerve cells have multiple receptors. Agonists can be "selective" in that they will bind to some receptors but not others.
- *Vascular:* Related to blood vessels.
- *Constrict:* Make smaller.
- *Trigeminal nerve:* The trigeminal nerve functions both as the chief nerve of sensation for the face and the motor nerve controlling the muscles of mastication (chewing). It gets its name from having three branches or divisions. The ophthalmic division carries sensations to the area around the eye, the maxillary carries sensations to the area of the up-

per jaw, and the mandibular division carries sensations to the area of the lower jaw.

Now let's dive in. Triptans are abortive medications. That means they're intended to abort a Migraine, cluster headache, or Migraine-like headache. To abort means to stop the headache or Migraine at its source, stopping the pain and all other symptoms of the attack. For purposes of explaining how triptans work, I'm going to talk about how they work on Migraine attacks, since that's their most common use.

Let's review what happens when we encounter a Migraine trigger. Migraineurs have overly excitable neurons (nerve cells that have the ability to transmit and receive nervous impulses) in our brains. When we encounter a trigger, those neurons fire in a wave across the brain, starting a series of events involving several centers of the brain, including the brain stem. The end of that series involves dilation or swelling of the blood vessels in the brain and the surrounding tissues, accompanied by inflammation of small arteries in the coverings of the brain. The headache of a Migraine attack, if there is one, is from sensory impulses transmitted by the nerves from these inflamed blood vessels and surrounding tissues transmitted to higher centers of the brain and experienced as pain.

Triptans are a class of medications called "selective serotonin receptor agonists." They go through the bloodstream to the brain, where they bind to serotonin receptors on cranial arteries and on the covering of the brain, working to constrict the blood vessels that have been dilated (made larger) by the Migraine process. They also activate serotonin receptors on terminals of the trigeminal nerve for inhibition of neuropeptide release and reduced transmission in trigeminal pain pathways. Each of the seven triptans has the potential to work somewhat differently and work for patients for whom other triptans didn't. Because they are *selective* serotonin receptor agonists, the different triptans bind to different serotonin receptors.

That allows them to act somewhat differently. Thus, if you've tried some of the triptans without success or with limited success, it's still worth trying the others.

Other Abortives

The first abortive medication was DHE-45 (dihydroergotamine) injections, introduced in the United States in 1945. DHE is also available in a nasal spray form called Migranal. Other ergotamine medications are available but not used as widely since the advent of triptans. Cafergot tablets and ergotamine suppositories are still used to some extent. Antinausea medications are often necessary with ergotamine medications.

For many cluster headache sufferers, inhaled medical oxygen has been found to be a fairly effective abortive therapy. Some Migraine sufferers have also reported at least partial relief with inhaled oxygen.

A new over-the-counter abortive is now available. The product is GelStat Migraine. Truthfully, my first reaction when I heard about it was skepticism. OTC products have never done much for me, and I didn't think this one would be any different. At this point, I have to take it all back and admit I was wrong. I find GelStat to be amazingly effective when used at the first sign of Migraine.

GelStat Migraine is a gel made of feverfew and ginger. Feverfew was first used for Migraine by the first-century Greek physician Dioscorides. Sir John Hill, an eighteenth-century English physician, wrote, "In the worst headaches, this herb exceeds whatever else is known." In much of Europe, feverfew was known as the "aspirin of the eighteenth century." How feverfew works for Migraine is not known. Ginger is native to India and China and has been an important part of traditional Chinese medicine for centuries.

Originally, feverfew was used by picking and chewing two fresh leaves. As a medication today, that's highly impractical. Most fever-few products contain dried and crushed leaves. The manufacturers of GelStat Migraine use fresh feverfew to make liquid feverfew, which is added to the gel base. Ginger is added to help with the nausea that is often a Migraine symptom. A side benefit of the ginger is that it helps cover the somewhat nasty taste of feverfew.

GelStat Migraine is packaged in the GelStat company's unique OraDose sublingual (under-the-tongue) delivery system. The Ora-Dose system is a small plastic vial with a tube that allows you to squeeze the contents under your tongue easily and quickly. You hold it under your tongue for sixty seconds before swallowing it. That allows the medication to be absorbed through the network of blood vessels under the tongue, which gives much faster absorption than medications that are swallowed and absorbed through the gastrointestinal tract. Medications passing through the digestive tract are absorbed slowly and are subject to a "first pass" effect in which many of the ingredients may be broken down by stomach acid or metabolized by the liver rather than producing the desired effect. Products absorbed sublingually enter the bloodstream directly and can start working within minutes.

GelStat doesn't work for me every time, but it does work 50–75 percent of the time. In a clinical trial conducted by Dr. Curtis P. Schreiber and Dr. Roger K. Cady of Springfield, Missouri, the following results emerged:

- 48 percent of participants were pain-free two hours after treatment of Migraine during mild pain.
- 83 percent were pain-free or had only mild pain two hours after treatment.
- Migraine-associated symptoms were absent two hours after treatment in 53 percent of participants.
- 41 percent preferred GelStat to their pre-study medication or felt it was equal to it.

■ Four subjects reported side effects. Three disliked the taste; one experienced transient burning under the tongue.

As with anything, you won't know if GelStat works for you unless you try it. However, even though it's made of "natural" ingredients, remember that such natural ingredients are where society got our first drugs. So discuss it with your doctor before trying this or any OTC product. For those of us who can't take triptans, GelStat is a welcome addition to our arsenal.

Other medications that aren't classified as abortives can, under the right circumstances, be effective as abortives. These are usually encountered in the emergency room or a headache and Migraine clinic. Depacon, which is a form of Depakote, usually used as a Migraine preventive, can be injected intravenously as a Migraine abortive. Intravenous magnesium will also sometimes abort a Migraine. Other medications that can be used include antinausea medications such as Compazine, Phenergan, and Reglan; antihistamines such as Benadryl; and anesthesia adjuncts such as Droperidol. In these circumstances, they're generally administered in injections, often in combinations.

Abortives for Children and Adolescents

If you look at the labeling and prescribing information for the triptans and ergotamine medications, you'll find it says they're not recommended for patients under the age of eighteen. In the report of the American Academy of Neurology Quality Standards Subcommittee and the Practice Committee of the Child Neurology Society discussed in the previous chapter, it was stated: "Sumatriptan (Imitrex/Imigran) nasal spray is effective and should be considered for the acute treatment of Migraine attacks in adolescents (over 12)."

Many doctors also prescribe some of the triptans for adolescents thirteen and older, unless they're exceptionally small for their age or have other health issues. If your child is under eighteen, and the doctor prescribes a triptan, discuss it with the doctor if it concerns you. Conversely, if the doctor doesn't prescribe a triptan, and you want to discuss the possibility, don't hesitate to approach the subject.

GelStat is also an option for children and adolescents. Again, talk with their doctor before giving it to them.

Summary

It's important to understand the difference between abortive medications and pain relievers. Pain relievers simply mask the pain for the period of time of their action. If your Migraine attack is over when the pain reliever wears off, that simply means it ran its course while you were under the effects of the medication. It does *not* mean that the pain reliever was able to stop the Migraine attack. Abortive medications, however, do work in the brain to stop Migraine attacks at their source. They stop the chain of events occurring in the brain that produce the symptoms of the Migraine attack. Abortive medications can also be effective for cluster headaches and Migraine-like headaches such as some post-traumatic headaches and new daily persistent headache.

14

Emergency Care and Pain Management

Anyone with Migraine disease or chronic headaches of any kind should have an emergency plan for times when regular treatments don't give relief. We have no way of knowing, let alone controlling, when a headache or Migraine will strike. Simple math tells us they're more likely to strike when our doctors are not in their offices. Most doctors aren't in their offices for a full 40-hour week, but let's work with a 40-hour week anyway. A full week is 168 hours. That leaves 128 hours of that week when our doctors are not in their offices for us to call them. That's nearly 70 percent of the time. This is exactly why we must be educated and able to make some treatment decisions for ourselves. It's also why that backup plan needs to be in place for times when our regular treatments fail us.

We must talk to our doctors in advance about an emergency care plan:

▮ Is there an after-hours number to call if we need assistance?
▮ What do we do if we have a headache or Migraine and our normal medications don't work?

■ If the doctor doesn't have an after-hours number to call, and our headache or Migraine reaches a point where we need care, is there a particular emergency room they recommend?

■ If we have to go to the emergency room, do they have advice for how to get the best treatment?

One element of a backup plan is called "rescue meds." Rescue meds are medications to be taken if and when the medications we normally take for our headaches and Migraines don't work. For those of us who use abortives, rescue meds are often pain medications. Sometimes rescue meds are a pain medication along with an antinausea medication. Essentially, if abortives fail, we have to resort to pain management if our headache or Migraine is still manageable enough to handle on our own at home.

If the emergency room is their recommendation for after-hours problems, ask your doctor to complete an Emergency Treatment Request and Information form. You'll find an example of this form at the end of this chapter and can print or download one from www.HelpForHeadaches.com/lwfiles/emergency-forms.htm. This form confirms your diagnosis, lists your current preventive and acute medications, and allows your doctor to suggest emergency treatment. In hopes of cutting through the unfortunate suspicions often encountered in ERs by those of us with invisible illnesses, the form also states that we are not substance abusers or "drug seekers." I'll be honest with you. There have been cases where these forms have been extremely helpful. There have also been cases where the ER doctors refused even to look at them. You simply won't know until you try. There's also a second form for us to fill out in advance. It has all the information that the registration clerk will need and saves us having to think about it when our head is pounding.

We need to be prepared for headache and Migraine emergencies in every way possible. Do you live alone? Even if you don't live alone, is someone generally available to take you to the doctor or emergency room if necessary? Plan ahead for this. We have no business driving ourselves under these circumstances. Not only is it unsafe for us and others on the roads, but people who have been in accidents caused by others have ended up in trouble themselves because they were driving after taking pain medications. Medications aren't the only reason for not driving. Pain slows our reflexes and dulls our concentration. There are many reasons not to drive during a headache or Migraine. Be safe first. If there are times when there's nobody home to help you get to the doctor or emergency room, check the availability of neighbors, friends, and family. If that's not an option, learn about taxi services in your area. If you have children, know whom you can call to watch them. Especially if you have children, it can be helpful to make an emergency event list. This can also be especially helpful if your children are old enough to help you a bit. List phone numbers you may need and things you need to remember to do or take with you:

- phone number of someone to take you to the doctor or emergency room
- phone number of someone to watch your children
- reminder to take list of all medications you have taken that day
- reminder to take insurance card with you
- reminder to take doctor's emergency form with you
- anything else you need to remember

Remember, we can minimize the impact of emergencies by planning ahead and organizing for them. The less we have to do and remember at the time, the less frantic we and everyone around us are likely to be. With everything else taken care of, we can concentrate on getting the medical care we need to get our headache or Migraine attack treated and feel better.

Pain Management

Even with all the preventives and abortives available to us today, there will be occasions when the appropriate treatment, even if just for a short time, is pain management. While trying to develop an effective preventive regimen, we may need relief. If we use abortives but limit their use to two or three days a week to avoid rebound, that leaves other days when we may need treatment. For times such as these, our doctors may prescribe various types of medications, including prescription pain medications. If you're taking prescription pain medications, please don't take over-the-counter pain medications also unless you discuss it with your doctor. The prescription medications often contain some of the same ingredients as the OTC medications (acetaminophen, for example), and you could accidentally take too much.

If you take OTC pain medications instead of prescription pain medications, please pay careful attention to and follow the recommended limits on the labels. OTC medications are every bit as potentially dangerous as prescription medications and should be treated accordingly.

Tip: If you're taking OTC Migraine medications, you may be able to save some money. When the manufacturers of Excedrin Migraine, Advil Migraine, and Motrin Migraine went to the FDA for approval to market their regular products for Migraine disease, they had to make changes in the labeling to indicate the recommended dosage for Migraine. They also made packaging changes and started packaging the same products under two names. The manufacturer's suggested retail prices for the original and Migraine products are the same. However, some stores are charging more for the Migraine products. Also, in the cases of Excedrin and Motrin, there are generic store brands that contain exactly the same ingredients but sell for lower prices. In other words:

- Excedrin Migraine = Extra Strength Excedrin = generic store brand
- Motrin Migraine = Motrin IB = generic store brand
- Advil Migraine = Advil LiquiGels

Another time when pain medications and pain management can come into play is for that extremely small percentage of people with chronic headaches or chronic Migraine for whom effective preventive regimens haven't been found. A good headache and Migraine specialist will work either directly with the patient or with the patient and a pain management specialist to devise a pain management regimen that improves his or her quality of life and offers at least some pain-free time. Since advancements are made in prevention all the time, it's important that anyone who falls into this category maintain a relationship with his or her headache and Migraine specialist. We never know when something might come along to change that situation for the better.

All of this has its place in good headache and Migraine management:

Headache Migraine management should have six parts:

1. Education.
2. Trigger identification and management: identifying what brings on your headaches or Migraine attacks and learning how to manage those triggers.
3. A good preventive regimen.
4. Appropriate abortives (medications that actually stop a Migraine attack rather than just masking the pain).
5. An emergency plan and pain management for times when abortives fail.
6. A strong support system.

Emergency Treatment Request and Information

Below is information that may assist you in treating my patient: _____

_____

for this severe Migraine episode. As you know, Migraine is a genetic neurological disease. Some episodes can require treatment beyond the medications the patient currently has for administration at home. Please note that this patient is neither a substance abuser nor a "drug seeker" but may need narcotic medications and other assistance to treat this episode.

Patient information:

Diagnosis: _____ Date of diagnosis: _____

Current preventive medication(s): _____

Current abortives and/or pain medication(s): _____

_____

Suggested treatment(s) for this patient in an emergency situation: _____

_____

Thank you for treating my patient. It is often very difficult for Migraine patients to receive adequate care offered with dignity and respect because of others who go to emergency departments and after-hours care facilities feigning symptoms to obtain narcotics. I assure you such is not the case with this patient.

Signature _____ Date _____

_____

Doctor's name, printed _____

Office Address _____

Office Phone_____

© Teri Robert 2005   www.HelpForHeadaches.com

Emergency Treatment Request and Information

Below is information that may assist you in treating my patient: _____

_____

for this severe cluster headache episode. As you know, cluster headaches are a serious, episodic neurological disorder. Some episodes can require treatment beyond the medications the patient currently has for administration at home. Please note that this patient is neither a substance abuser nor a "drug seeker" but may need narcotic medications and other assistance to treat this episode.

Patient information:

Diagnosis: _____Date of diagnosis: _____

Current preventive medication(s): _____

Current abortives and/or pain medication(s): _____

_____

Suggested treatment(s) for this patient in an emergency situation: _____

_____

Thank you for treating my patient. It is often very difficult for cluster headache patients to receive adequate care offered with dignity and respect because of others who go to emergency departments and after-hours care facilities feigning symptoms to obtain narcotics. I assure you such is not the case with this patient.

Signature _____ Date _____

_____

Doctor's name, printed _____

Office Address _____

Office Phone_____

© Teri Robert 2005   www.HelpForHeadaches.com

Emergency Treatment Registration Information

I am experiencing extreme head pain resulting from a Migraine attack. I am not a "drug seeker" and have brought a form from my doctor verifying my diagnosis and treatment information.

Full Name _____

Address _____

City_____State _____Zip Code_____

Home Phone_____Office Phone_____

Employer_____

Emergency Contact _____Relationship _____Phone Number _____

Treatment Information: On a scale of 1–10, I currently rate my pain at _____.

To treat this Migraine attack, I have taken these medications:

Medication _____Dosage _____Time Taken _____

Medication _____Dosage _____Time Taken _____

Medication _____Dosage _____Time Taken _____

Other Medications: _____

Allergies: _____

© Teri Robert 2004, 2005 · www.HelpForHeadaches.com

Emergency Treatment Registration Information

I am experiencing extreme head pain resulting from a cluster headache. I am not a "drug seeker" and have brought a form from my doctor verifying my diagnosis and treatment information.

Full Name _____

Address _____

City_____State _____Zip Code_____

Home Phone_____Office Phone_____

Employer_____

Emergency Contact _____Relationship _____Phone Number _____

Treatment Information: On a scale of 1–10, I currently rate my pain at _____.

To treat this cluster headache, I have taken these medications:

Medication_____Dosage _____Time Taken _____

Medication_____Dosage _____Time Taken _____

Medication_____Dosage _____Time Taken _____

Other Medications: _____

Allergies: _____

© Teri Robert 2004, 2005   www.HelpForHeadaches.com

15

Complementary Therapies

Some people would say "alternative therapies," but I prefer "complementary therapies." The term *alternative therapies* seems to indicate that you choose one type or the other. That's not necessary. These therapies can work quite well in concert with more traditional therapies. Thus the term *complementary therapies*. They complement one another.

Aromatherapy

Aromatherapy is quite often used for headaches and Migraine. You may find that even if it doesn't actually relieve your pain, it will help you relax. The benefits of relaxation during a headache or Migraine are enormous. Aromatherapy can also do a great deal to relieve the nausea that so often accompanies Migraine attacks. There are many forms of aromatherapy: candles, incense, bath products, essential oils, and more. The most concentrated and perhaps most therapeutic is the use of essential oils. Essential oils can be used in diffusers to release their aroma into the air or applied to the skin. It's important to remember that these oils are very concentrated and, with the possible exception of lavender, should not be applied directly to the skin without first being mixed with a basic oil (called a carrier oil). Oils commonly used as carrier oils include sweet almond, apricot kernel, and fractionated coconut. There is a commercial product named Migrastick that combines lavender and peppermint oils in a small, 3-mL/0.1-ounce roll-on bottle that sells for about $6. It's recommended for massaging lightly at the temples. It is not recommended for pregnant or breast-feeding women or people with epilepsy. If you already work with essential oils or would like to, you might prefer to make your own. That lets you customize the oils and blend a similar product less expensively. Roll-on bottles are available from many aromatherapy supply companies. Some of the essential oils most commonly recommended for headache and Migraine include lavender, peppermint, chamomile, clary sage, melissa, jasmine, and rosemary. The peppermint is especially good for relieving nausea. These same oils, individually or in different combinations, can also be used in a diffuser.

Acupressure

Acupressure is an ancient Asian method of finger pressure massage that targets twelve invisible energy channels called "meridians" throughout the body. These meridians are used in various forms of traditional Eastern medicine. Blockage in the flow of chi (vital energy) is thought to cause pain. Releasing chi promotes wellness. Acupressure was used in China as early as 2000 BC, before acupuncture. Acupressure is very similar to shiatsu massage. It can be self-administered (once learned) in some cases or administered by a professional. Depending on how blocked the energy is, more than one session may be required to see significant relief. Once relief is achieved, regular sessions are recommended as a form of prevention and to maintain overall health.

Acupuncture

Originating in China more than two thousand years ago, acupuncture is one of the oldest, most commonly used medical procedures in the world. In traditional Chinese medicine, one of the major assumptions is that health is achieved by keeping the body in a balanced state. That means a balance of the two forces yin and yang. An imbalance leads to a blockage in the flow of chi along the twelve pathways of the body known as meridians. There are more than two thousand acupuncture points on the human body connecting the meridians. It's said that acupuncture works with the neurotransmitters serotonin and norepinephrine to block transmission of pain and produce the body's pain-relieving hormones, endorphins.

In the United Kingdom, researchers recruited 401 adult patients with at least two headaches per month for a study of the benefits of acupuncture for chronic headache. For three months, patients received either their usual care alone or their usual care plus as many as twelve acupuncture treatments. At the end of twelve months, the study showed:

- There was a 34 percent reduction in headaches in the acupuncture group; 16 percent in the control group.
- Acupuncture group patients experienced twenty-two fewer days of headache yearly than control group patients.
- Acupuncture group patients used 15 percent less medication than control group patients.
- Acupuncture group patients made 25 percent fewer family doctor visits than control group patients.

▌ Acupuncture group patients took 15 percent fewer sick days than control group patients.

Biofeedback

Biofeedback can be used on its own or in combination with medications or other therapies. Children usually become adept at biofeedback more quickly than adults do, but with patience, most adults can master it also. Biofeedback operates on the premise that we have a natural potential and ability to influence certain autonomic (involuntary) functions. Computers and computerized monitors are used to teach biofeedback. Once mastered, it can be used anywhere, at any time, with no need for any equipment. Several types of equipment are used to learn biofeedback. Three of the most common are the following:

▌ EMG (electromyogram) biofeedback is taught using an EMG machine, which measures electrical activity in the muscles through electrodes attached to the skin with adhesive patches. For purposes of biofeedback, the muscles most commonly used are those of the forehead, jaw, and upper shoulders. During a biofeedback training session, electrodes are placed on muscles in those three areas, and the patient concentrates on relaxing. The EMG machine can be programmed to produce a tone or turn on a light for each muscle group in which tension is detected.

▌ Temperature biofeedback employs a temperature sensor that is attached to the patient's finger or foot. When a person is stressed or anxious, blood is redirected to muscles and inner organs, and skin temperature drops. Again, the sensor is attached to a computer, and either a tone or light can be used to signal changes in skin temperature.

▌ Galvanic skin response may sound familiar; it's also used as a "lie detector." Through electrodes attached to the skin, a very slight (unnoticeable) charge is run through the skin. The machine the electrodes lead to measures changes in the water and salt in your sweat gland ducts. This is an effective measurement because heightened emotions increase your skin's conductivity.

The immediate physical goals of biofeedback may vary. The goal may be to relax muscles, slow and regulate breathing, or learn to redirect blood to the hands to warm them. Biofeedback is commonly paired with relaxation training, meditation, or visualization techniques. The therapeutic goals vary as well. Some doctors recommend temperature biofeedback for Migraineurs, working on the theory that redirecting blood to the hands to warm them will pull blood from the head and relieve Migraines. Some recommend it for lowering blood pressure. It is often recommended simply for relaxation to lead to better overall health.

Crystal Therapy

One of the basic principles behind crystal therapy lies in the theory that different crystals or stones have different vibrations. An interaction between the vibration of the crystal and the vibration of the person triggers healing responses. Some people believe that crystals were created by God and can have healing properties just as herbs and minerals do. They reason that if we grind up minerals and ingest them, why not use whole stones and crystals for healing effects?

In my reading, the crystal I've seen most associated with healing/preventing headaches and Migraine is amethyst. Others include cat's-eye, dioptase, magnesite, smoky quartz, and sugilite. When using crystals for headache or Migraine prevention, you should carry or wear one with you and sleep with one at the head of your bed. There have been no clinical trials using crystals. When I was introduced to these theories, I figured, "Why not?" I got some amethyst, put one at the head of my bed, and began wearing one on a chain around my neck. There was some decrease in my Migraine frequency. Can it be proven to be attributable to the amethyst? No, but even my Migraine specialist can't say it isn't. So it hasn't replaced any of my medications, but it may be helping some. If there isn't a shop near you to buy crystals, check online. There are many online sources, including eBay. Do some comparison shopping so you don't pay too much.

Massage Therapy

In general, massage therapy can be good for overall health, and anything that's good for overall health helps us with headaches and Migraine. Massage improves blood flow, increases the oxygenation of blood, helps with muscle relaxation, and stimulates the production of endorphins. When we get into specifics, massage therapy tends to be more helpful in cases of tension-type headaches or Migraines that are triggered by tension-type headaches. For true massage therapy, it's best to locate a registered massage therapist. If recommended by your doctor, it may even be covered by your medical insurance. There are various forms of massage therapy, including Swedish massage, deep tissue massage, and hydrotherapy.

Meditation

Meditation is another technique toward better overall health. It's also a way to sometimes mentally escape pain. Meditation is intended to achieve a state of balance and is often associated with the practitioner's personal spiritualism. It's been described as "a path to a higher state of consciousness." There are several types of meditation—Buddhist, transcendental, Zen, Taoist, primordial sound, and others. Most people start with the one that makes them most comfortable, then adapt it to make it their own.

Relaxation

It's amazing how tense some of us are even when we think we're relaxed. I have a friend who, when we're spending an evening together, will put his hand on my back and ask if I'm comfortable and relaxed. The first time he did that, when I said, "Yes," he raised an eyebrow. He then proceeded to rub the tension out of about a dozen spots on my shoulders and upper back. Ouch! He truly did me a favor by showing me how much of the day's tension was being held in those muscles even though I had thought I was quite relaxed. I was on a week-long business trip in his hometown and hadn't taken my relaxation CD with me. Although I had missed my daily routine of listening to the CD, it hadn't been an especially stressful week. But I had spent several hours that afternoon on the telephone helping Migraineurs who were having severe problems. When we started talking, we both realized that their problems were still on my mind (and probably in my back and shoulders). That served to reinforce the advice of my Migraine specialist, who recommends that I listen to my favorite relaxation tape or CD every day, regardless of how I feel. Now I keep one in my luggage. You don't have to have a recording to use relaxation techniques. You can manage on your own by concentrating on relaxing your body and letting go of tensions. I find that difficult. After a few minutes, my mind is wandering back to what I was doing or what I should do tomorrow. With a recording, I'm far more likely to stay on track. There are innumerable relaxation recordings from which to choose. I favor *Effortless Relaxation* by Steven Halpern, Ph.D. Dr. Halpern is an educator, composer, author, and recording artist of international acclaim. After listening to his CD, I tracked him down for an interview and asked about the unique qualities of his music. He explained that he liked to keep the tempos no faster than the relaxed heartbeat people will be trying to achieve. He also composes without repeating patterns or melodies in his relaxation music, because repetition only makes the brain automatically wait and listen to recognize them.

I find the relaxation program to be an excellent daily tool for overall health and a big help when I have a Migraine. During a Migraine attack, after I've taken medication, it will often help me relax enough to fall asleep.

PART THREE

Support and Empowerment

16

Support: As Important as Good Medical Care

TRUE STORY #1: THE HUGE NEED FOR SUPPORT

Desperate and alone. Well, I am alive again after another day of hell. It always surprises me that there is life after the ER. I pray so hard for death when I am in the throes of a cluster/Migraine. (Period started today, so there's my trigger.) I vomited and dry-heaved for a solid ten hours yesterday, and when I say this, I am sure someone else has had to experience this. . . . I mean, I could not get a breath in between, and honest to God I prayed for death.

The panic and horror never ceases to amaze me. You would think that I would be used to this. But each time feels like the first, and I swear I can never go through it again and keep my sanity . . . yet I do. My teachings in enlightenment and power of the self go right out the window, and breathing and meditation are lost somewhere. (Maybe the IV interferes?) Does anyone else turn into a screaming banshee the way that I do? I beg and plead and yell and run in circles, banging my head off the wall! I am embarrassed as all heck after the fact, but I seem to lose total control.

Yesterday, a man that I just started seeing had the pleasure of watching me go through this as he removed basin after basin of vomit from me. I'll bet that is the end of that! I just couldn't bear to be alone and he offered, so. . . . What a dummy I am. I wish I could just give all of you a hug, and please know how much the support of this place means. I do love you all.

The need for support is twofold. There are the practical concerns of having someone to help when you need it. Just as important, perhaps even more so, is the very human need for acceptance, understanding, and emotional support. In addition to the physical pain, headache disorders and Migraine disease come with a wide range of emotional issues:

▌ *Isolation:* We can easily end up feeling cut off from the rest of the world when we're in pain and unable to get out and do the things we're used to doing. This is especially true of people who are used to being active.

▌ *Guilt:* It's easy to start feeling guilty for missing family events or not getting done the things we usually do. What's more, if our child inherits Migraine disease, we can really get the guilts for that reason, too. That gets tied in to our sense of self-worth, and it can start slipping. Headache disorders and Migraines can be even more effective than a mother at inducing guilt trips. (Yes, I can say that. I have two children.)

TRUE STORY #2: UNDESERVED GUILT
I've passed it down: It is 1:47 a.m. as I write this post. I have been at the Children's Hospital with my thirteen-year-old daughter since 8:15 p.m. She got her first Migraine tonight, on top of the flu. Of all the things I had to pass down to her,

this is by far one of the worst. I could do nothing but watch helplessly as she lay there in too much pain to even cry as she looked at me and begged me to make the pain go away. She spent most of last night vomiting, so she was dehydrated as well as sick and in pain. She got a liter of saline and this drug that is supposed to be for controlling violent nausea but has a side effect of making Migraines go away. She is in her bed now, and I keep checking on her to make sure she is okay.

I feel so guilty right now. I am smart enough to know that I did nothing to make this happen, it's genetic, but it doesn't stop the guilt and feeling like the worst parent in the world. I love her so much, I would willingly give my life for her. If that is what would make her pain stop, I'd do it.

■ *Anger:* Anger can get directed at the illness, at ourselves, at our doctors, at life in general. It can also sometimes get misdirected toward those around us. There can be another way anger rears its ugly head. If you think your spouse or significant other is angry with you about your episodes, you may be correct that he or she is angry but wrong about the reason for the anger. We tend to want to "fix things" when we love someone. Those around us can feel totally helpless to do anything at all for us, let alone fix things. Sometimes what we perceive as anger toward us is actually anger toward the situation and the illness. If you feel you're in this type of situation, sit down and talk with the other person. Tell him or her that they seem angry. Ask with whom or what they're angry. We can't begin to address such a problem until we begin communicating.

■ *Grief:* Think about it. As strange as it may sound, if we don't make progress in our treatment after a while, and we're incapacitated for some time, we can start grieving for the life we had and now feel we've lost. We can start feeling some of the same emotions and go through some of the same stages of grief that we do when we lose a loved one.

■ *Depression:* This one gets tricky. If we feel depressed, it's important to make notes and see if the depression deepens and lightens according to how we feel physically and talk to our doctor about it. It will need to be determined if it's an emotional depression resulting from the upheaval the headaches and/or Migraines have created in our lives or if it's clinical depression, which is a disease. It's not fully understood yet exactly what the link is between Migraine disease and clinical depression, but 47 percent of Migraineurs also experience clinical depression. Depression's prevalence in the general population is only 17 percent. Those statistics show an undeniable link.

■ *Fear:* Fear is a big one, and it takes many forms. People are afraid of being alone, afraid of being a burden, afraid a Migraine attack will cause a stroke, even afraid of the next Migraine attack.

TRUE STORIES #3 AND #4: MIGRAINE ATTACKS AND FEAR

Terrified by Migraine without the pain. For the first time in almost twenty years, I have had my period without the throbbing, gut-wrenching whirlwind of pain I always got. I was terrified. Unfortunately, without the pain I noticed more of the other symptoms that have always accompanied my Migraines but weren't such a big deal because the throbbing explosions of pain going off in my head were all too consuming to really take notice of these other things. Well, I'm noticing now and I like it even less than the pain.

I certainly wasn't prepared to be pain-free. I had gotten so used to the pain, I actually found myself anticipating it. Of course, when the pain didn't start but all the other auras asso-

ciated with the Migraine did, I panicked. I called the doctor in hysterics because I thought I was having a stroke instead of a Migraine. Helena at the Jefferson Headache Center was an angel. She calmed me down enough for me to realize that it was still the Migraine without the pain.

Fear of Migraines. *I find that I am sometimes more immobilized by my fear of the next Migraine than the Migraine itself. I spend more time in the safe, dimly lit, soft acoustics of my bedroom (cave) than venturing out into the bright, overstimulating world. My life-of-fear exists in between expensive, hard-to-get-approved Imitrex injections. What kind of life is this? All the failed preventive pharmacology, all the supplements and altered diets, all the canceled social plans, missed work. . . . When will it end?*

When will I really be Migraine-free—or at least free of the fear?

By now, I'm sure you can see where this is leading. Our medical team helps us with our medical treatment needs, but that certainly doesn't address the basic human emotional needs that can be met by a good support system.

Give it a bit of thought. Yes, good medical care is vital. However, good support is just as vital. Without support, there might well be times when we couldn't get to the doctor to get medical care or times there would be nobody to watch our children while we went to the doctor. There could be days when we were flat on our backs in bed and nobody was around to help us. We have practical, functional needs that are met by a good support system.

That very same support system can, at times, be all that stands between us and hitting rock bottom emotionally. As with other parts of life, it's often the seemingly small things that can make the biggest difference.

17

When Those Close to You Don't Understand

TRUE STORY #5: LACKING UNDERSTANDING AT HOME

"I hope the new med doesn't work"! Yep, that's what my amazing boyfriend said to me the other night. Needless to say, I didn't talk to him the rest of the night!

I've been suffering from the same Migraine since early July and was just put on Epival (Depakote) after a bad reaction with the Topamax. Well, after a week on my full dose, there has been no change. My boyfriend asked me about it and then, knowing some of the possible side effects, said that "I almost hope it doesn't work 'cause I don't want you to be 250 pounds"! I flipped. I asked him if he would rather see me like this, in bed in the dark, every day instead. It just hurt so much because he of all people knows how hard a time I'm having! Nothing is getting rid of the pain fully, so far no success with preventives, I'm in hell every day without fail. I talked to him later, and he said he didn't mean for it to come out the way it did, which I believe because that isn't the person he is; but it still did.

Yesterday he came home from work and apologized again, I think he thought about it all day and really realized what he'd said, and how it made me feel. I just lost twenty pounds I gained from amitriptyline, and I don't want to gain it, either, but if it works, it works!! Just wanted to vent, as it hurt, even if he didn't mean it that way!

Many people with problem headaches and Migraines say, "Unless a person gets these, they just don't understand!" There's a certain amount of truth in that, but I hold out hope that education can prevail in many instances when no one seems to understand what you're going through. There are some factors that contribute to this lack of understanding:

- For too long, not much was known about chronic headaches and Migraine disease. As with most anything about which little is known, myths and stereotypes developed. It's difficult to dispel them. That has to be done through education. The general public has limited exposure to such education, and doctors don't always stay as up-to-date as we would like.
- Migraine is an invisible disease. Chronic headaches are an invisible disorder as well. We don't have the outward symptoms of disease or treatment as do those who have cancer, heart disease, diabetes, or epilepsy. We don't have casts on broken bones or bandages on outer wounds from headaches or Migraine.
- For someone who has never experienced severe, chronic headaches or a Migraine attack, it's extraordinarily difficult to comprehend the level of pain and disability that it causes.

Family

True Story #6: What About the Spouse?

Spouses and Migraines. Has anyone ever had problems with their spouses not understanding Migraines? Mine sometimes thinks I make this up because it happens so often. I ask this: "Why would anyone even want to act a Migraine?" Or should I say, How would you? I can throw up, cry because of the pain (which I know doesn't help). How can I get through to him and make him understand what it feels like? I do feel very emotional anyway because of all the meds I'm on. I just don't need this too! I hope someone has answers for these questions, 'cause I can't take this anymore.

In many ways, it's most difficult when the people who don't understand are family members, especially family members within your own household. These are the people we love, with whom we have the most contact, and who impact our lives the most. Their lack of understanding can be devastating. But what can you do?

- If you have these people in your life, have you taken any of them to your doctor with you? I've seen that help family members understand better. There's just something about being in the doctor's office when you're discussing your condition that makes it more real to them. Especially if your doctor knows the situation in advance, accompanying you to a doctor's appointment can be a turning point for a family member.
- Have you shared your books and other educational materials with them? If not, give it a try. Right now, take this book, go back to the earlier chapters that explain your type

of head pain, and go over some of the information with them. Show them how your condition is different from a "plain vanilla" headache. If you want some additional material, you can go online and print some letters I've written to help educate people. You'll find them at www. HelpForHeadaches.com/lwfiles/letters.htm. If you don't have Internet access, stop by the public library. Most libraries now have computers with Internet access that you can use. Here's an example of those materials:

A Letter to Share with Family, Friends, and Co-Workers
RE: Understanding Migraine Disease and Migraineurs

If you're reading this, someone close to you is a Migraineur, someone diagnosed with Migraine, a recognized neurological disease. Migraine is one of the most misunderstood, under-diagnosed, and undertreated of all diseases. Unless you've experienced the pain of Migraine yourself, it is very difficult to comprehend. It is not an exaggeration to say that some people have committed suicide to escape the pain. In addition to the extreme head pain, Migraine can be accompanied by other symptoms, including nausea, vomiting, dizziness, extreme sensitivity to light and sound, temporary loss of vision, inability to concentrate, difficulty in speaking/finding the right words, depression, panic attacks, and far more. The slightest movement can cause such pain that Migraineurs have described it as "an ice pick in my eye," "my head breaking into pieces," and "my brain exploding." To put it plainly, Migraine can be absolutely devastating.

Here are some points about Migraine disease that you should know:

■ *Based on the most recent U.S. census statistics, Migraine disease affects approximately 32.5 million people in the United States alone.*

■ *Migraines are* not *headaches. Migraine is a* neurological disease, *similar in some ways to epilepsy. The head pain of a Migraine attack is only one symptom of an episode of Migraine disease, just as a seizure is only one symptom of an episode of epilepsy.*

■ *Migraine disease is* not *a psychological disorder. The disease and all its symptoms are neurological in origin and very, very real. Migraineurs are not neurotic, lazy, "high-strung," overly emotional, or faking. They are in very real pain and physical distress.*

■ Not all doctors have the experience and knowledge to treat Migraine properly. Finding the right doctor to treat Migraine is one of the most important, and sometimes most difficult, steps in treatment.

■ *There is* no cure *for Migraine. Most Migraineurs, with the help of a qualified doctor, can find preventive regimens that will prevent many, but not all, Migraine attacks.*

■ *Migraine abortive medications such as Imitrex, Zomig, Maxalt, Amerge, Axert, Frova, DHE, and Migranal do not work for all Migraineurs. It is sometimes very difficult to find medications that will relieve the pain and other symptoms of a Migraine attack.*

■ Migraine attacks can be dangerous. *If the pain of an attack lasts more than seventy-two hours with less than four pain-free hours while awake, it is termed "status Migrainous" and puts the sufferer at increased risk for stroke.* A Migraineur in status Migrainous needs immediate medical attention.

■ A Migraine attack can actually be fatal. *An otherwise*

healthy twenty-one-year-old member of our community died of a Migrainous stroke in November, 2001. According to the National Migraine Association, more people die each year from Migrainous stroke than are killed by handguns.

■ *Migraine disease can be* disabling *for some Migraineurs to the extent that they qualify for disability income or qualify for Americans with Disability Act provisions. There are many whose disease is so severe that doctors are unable to control the attacks, and the Migraineur is unable to work or participate in "normal" daily activities.* When a Migraine attack strikes, most Migraineurs desperately need a dark, quiet place to lie down.

■ *Migraine attacks can be triggered by many things:*
  - **Perfumes and fragrances** *from other sources are a very common Migraine trigger. If you live or work with a Migraineur, please refrain from wearing fragrances around him or her.*
  - **Bright and/or flickering lights***, especially fluorescent lighting—some Migraineurs need to wear sunglasses, even inside.*
  - *Many* **foods** *can be triggers, especially foods prepared with MSG.*
  - *Loud noises and crowded places can also be triggers.*
  - **Changes in weather** *are triggers for many Migraineurs.*
  - *Cigarette smoke, exhaust fumes.*
  - **Each Migraineur's triggers vary.** *There are many other potential triggers. This list is just a beginning.*

The Migraineurs in your life need your help and understanding. They need you to realize that they cannot help being ill, they are not "having headaches for attention," and they are sometimes unable to care for themselves. If they need medical attention, they need someone to take them and be with them. As well as being extremely painful physically, Migraine can be devastating emotionally and to relationships and careers. Since the disease is so misunderstood, Migraineurs often feel alone, isolated, and desolate. They also often feel guilty because they are not able to "be there" for their family and friends as much as they want to be and because they may have to miss days of work. The Migraineurs you know need not only your help with getting their medicines and any medical care they may need; they need your moral support every bit as badly. A good, solid support system is as important to Migraineurs as their health care teams. You are very important to them. That's why it's important that you understand Migraine.

Sincerely,
Teri Robert

▋ If it's your spouse who seems not to understand, sit down and have a conversation with him or her to see if lack of understanding is really the problem. In many cases, it's more complicated than that. Spouses who love us tend to want to fix things for us. When they can't, it can become so frustrating to them that it comes across as not understanding or being less caring than they are.

Here's a point that's often overlooked: When one family member has an illness or disease, there are times when the whole family, especially the spouse, needs support.

■ If nothing else seems to be working, consider family counseling. Your doctor may very well be able to recommend someone to help you with this.

Our Illness Becomes a Family Illness

As much as we're hurting and need support, there's something else we have to consider. When one person in a family has an illness or disease, everyone might as well have it because they're so strongly affected by it. This makes it important to try to have support from outside your immediate family.

TRUE STORY #7: WHAT ABOUT OUR CHILDREN?

Real or sympathetic? Here's a new wrinkle in my headache situation. The other day, I told my son I needed to lie down because I had a headache, and he could watch a video. He looked at me and said, "But, Mommy, my head hurts, too!" I can usually tell when this child doesn't feel well by how his eyes look, and they looked fine. I didn't know what to do, so I gave him his own little ice pack and let him lie down with me. When my husband came home, he told his daddy that he and Mommy had to go to bed with headaches. I'm going to make an appointment with his pediatrician, but do any of you think he could be pretending or talking himself into a headache because he isn't getting enough attention? I'd love to hear from any other moms if you've had this situation or even if you haven't.

This can especially affect children. That can present a special problem because some children, when they know a parent is ill, will hide their feelings. They may be afraid of making their parent feel worse. If old enough, they may not want to add to their parent's stress. The problem that's created is this: When a parent is ill, a child needs more attention. Unfortunately, this is usually when the parent is least able to give that extra attention.

Here are some suggestions for ways to reduce the stress our illness places on our children:

A great tip from a chronic Migraine sufferer: As my Migraines became more frequent, I started to see the effect on my children. My Migraines weren't robbing just me of normalcy, they were robbing my kids, too. What could I do to give them back some of that normalcy when I was in pain and in bed several days a week? I got my sister to go to work with me on this one. We got a big plastic storage chest and filled it with fun and educational things for the kids—puzzles, word games, coloring books, videos, and so on. Since I don't like prepackaged food for my kids, we hit the kitchen next. We made a huge pot of vegetable noodle soup the kids like and a large casserole with chicken, rice, and vegetables. When those were done, we packaged them in individual servings and put them in the freezer. At the grocery store, we got juice boxes and individual serving packages of snacks. Those we put in another plastic storage chest. Now the plastic storage chests are in a corner of our family room, and the freezer is kept stocked with nutritional meals for my kids. My son is old enough to get the food out and safely microwave it if I just can't do it. It even makes him feel good to do it for his sisters. Since the toys in the "Migraine chest" are only for those days, they don't get bored with them. I hope this will help other people, too.

▪ Most important, our children need to understand that our headaches and Migraine attacks are not their fault. There can be a tendency in children to think they caused anything bad that happens around them. It's essential now and for their future well-being that they not feel this way.

▌ We need to educate our children about Migraine disease and headaches. How we go about educating them will, of course, depend a lot upon their age. Some older children will do well with the same educational materials we use for ourselves and other adults. Younger children will need special care and attention. There is an excellent book, *Mama Lion's Migraine,* by Alden R. Carter, that is the best tool I've seen for educating young children about Migraine disease. It's not available commercially, but it is available from Pfizer as part of its "Understanding in a Box." You can request a free "Understanding in a Box" kit from its Web site, www.relpax.com.

▌ If they still take naps, and we need to lie down at a good time for them to take a nap, it can be very comforting for them to take their nap with us. It can be comforting for us, too!

▌ Find ways to let them help us. Most kids love to help. If you use ice packs, put them in a place in your freezer where your child can reach them. Then, ask your child to get one for you, even if you do feel up to getting it for yourself. Do the same thing with beverages and snacks you might want when you have a Migraine attack or headache.

▌ If possible, prepare in advance for quiet activities your children can do wherever you rest or sleep when you have a headache or Migraine attack. Coloring books, regular books (if they're old enough to read for themselves), sticker books, small dolls, quiet games, and other calm, quiet activities can allow them to stay in the room with you when you're resting. They feel safer, and they may even feel that they're watching over us just as we watch over them when they're not well. Depending on the arrangement of the room, you may even be able to set up a video or DVD for them to watch quietly.

- If it's not possible for your children to stay with you during an episode, or if they're older, plan in advance for activities to keep them occupied when you're not well.

- With older children, we need to take care not to let too much responsibility fall on them because of our illness. That can happen very easily, without our even realizing it's happening. There will be times when asking older children to do things we would normally be taking care of is unavoidable. That in itself is fine—as long as it doesn't happen too often. It can even make the older child feel as if he or she is helping and contributing to the family. We just need to be careful about how often it happens and remember to praise the child for his or her efforts.

- Above all, we need to tell our children the truth. Telling them we're tired or making other excuses will bite us in the rear later on. We're all born with what some people call natural empathy, a form of emotional communication. Since it's not recognized, trained, or nurtured, it generally just goes away as we grow up. *But,* that's how children know when something is wrong and when we're not telling them the truth. They may not say anything, but they know, and that affects how they grow up and how they deal with issues as adults. Also, we have enough problems with people who don't understand headaches and Migraines. Let's not contribute to yet another generation that doesn't understand.

Co-workers and Employers

True Story #8: When Co-workers Create Migraine Triggers

Perfume in the workplace: I have been through what you might call perfume hell as far as the workplace goes. I work in a sales-oriented company. They do community campaigns, public service announcements basically for various radio stations. I am the administrator there. Only nonsalesperson. One of the salespeople at the company, a woman who is one of the top producers, used to wear very strong aromatic perfumes. She can be very high-strung to start with, as well as having a major attitude to go with it. Anyway, there was a period of time I was proud of the fact that I was off any preventive Migraine medication. As soon as Denise walked into office, I swear I could smell her at ten paces, the effect was that intense. Before she entered the office I felt fine. As soon as she was in the office, it was as though I were part bloodhound. I could feel my sinuses clogging up; my nose felt really stuffy. Then I could feel a tight band around my head, became extremely dizzy, and literally felt like passing out. Needless to say, I had an appointment with the white bowl shortly after. This happened a couple of times, and I went over to her desk and asked to speak to her for a moment. I spoke to her in a nonconfrontational tone and asked her politely if she could refrain from wearing the perfume she had on. She knew I was a Migraine sufferer but just didn't understand how her perfume could be affecting me. The tone in her voice told me she had a problem with my even approaching her. I thought, "Here we go!" Unfortunately, Denise took this whole thing very personally and would not quit wearing *the perfume. Eventually I had to take up the issue with the owner of the company. It was either that or not be able to work.*

When you have chronic headaches or Migraine disease, holding down a job is difficult enough under the best of circumstances. Co-workers and employers who don't have a clue can make it unbearable. I know. Tell you something you don't know. Right? There's no right solution here, no right piece of advice to offer, because we're talking about people and personalities. Let's not give up, though! Here are some things that have worked:

▌ Obviously, you should always be pleasant toward your co-workers and employer. You also don't want to always be complaining about how awful you feel and how much pain you're enduring. However, being too good an actor can be to your detriment. Some of us have lived with pain for so long that we can force a smile and appear fairly "normal." If you're working with the public, that's going to be important, but don't push it too far with your co-workers or employers. It could backfire by giving them the impression that your pain isn't really all that bad and you're not really all that ill. So when it's just you and your co-workers and/or employer, I recommend neither the "I'm just fine" facade nor going for any dramatic effect. Your pain will show in your face and bearing, and that's just fine. The answer to the question "How are you?" can always be, "Making do," "Getting by," or something else similar that does not say "Fine" yet doesn't seem like a complaint.

▌ Divide and conquer! If one person at work understands, that person can often help with the others. We all know there's bound to be discussion of our condition among the other employees. If one person understands and is willing to help, you can provide that person with some basic educational materials so he or she knows some things to tell your other co-workers and perhaps even your boss. This is even better if the person who understands happens to be your boss.

■ Schedule a one-on-one conversation with your supervisor. Get yourself focused and your emotions under control before this session begins. It's often helpful to make notes of what you want to say in advance of this session. You can also take copies of educational materials with you. The attitude you want to achieve is that of someone who is calm and professional and in a problem-solving mode. Begin by thanking him or her for taking the time to meet with you. Unless it's totally absurd to do so, also thank him or her for the support he or she has given you. Let him or her know that you like your job, are good at it, are loyal to the company. Work in some good points about the company and staff. Then you can tell him or her that you have a medical condition that is very seldom well understood, and you'd like to work with him or her on that in order to reduce any stress it creates for you and anyone else there. Now— ready . . . set . . . educate! This is another time you can use the letters I referred to earlier when talking about family members who don't understand.

Obviously, there are no guarantees that those suggestions will solve any and all problems your headaches and Migraines help create at work. We can always hope! In chapter 20, we'll discuss our legal rights, including those applicable to our employment.

Friends

Teenage and young adult sufferers, especially, have told me their friends essentially quit coming around when they kept having to cancel plans to go out and do things. I can remember being their age and can well understand what they're saying. When headaches and Migraines are chronic, they can teach us a difficult life lesson. When reality stares us in the face, we find that most of us have far more acquaintances than true friends.

At whatever age, if your friends seem to stop calling as much because you've had to turn down some invitations, get creative. Invitations run both directions, so get on the phone and invite them to do something. If the activities you usually share are triggering activities for you, here's where a bit of creativity can enter the situation. Think "outside the box," as the expression goes. Look beyond the activities you usually share and find others you can share and mutually enjoy without triggering a headache or Migraine. You're taking the initiative here to invite them. Friends will appreciate that and should respond well to it.

Here's something else to consider. Social relationships with all their cues and miscues are complex to begin with. People tend to make them ridiculously complex by worrying about "socially acceptable," "politically correct," and myriad other dynamics that, quite bluntly, are foolish and unnecessary, especially among friends. Still, they're often there despite the fact that they tend to be far more destructive than constructive. Remember that, and take the high road. Don't underestimate your friends. Give them the benefit of the doubt and consider that contemporary society mixes things up sometimes. So before you give up on those you think have given up on you, talk with them about the problem. If you're not comfortable talking with them in person or by telephone, consider a letter or an e-mail. During your conversation or in your letter or e-mail, take the opportunity to let them know you have an illness that goes beyond headaches, and try to educate them. Teach them some of what you've learned about your headaches, Migraine disease, or both. Give them some of the statistics from earlier chapters of this book. If you want a bit of help, this is another time you can use the letters at www.HelpForHeadaches.com/lwfiles/letters.htm.

18

Building Your Support System

Support can come from many places. Let's start with the most obvious:

■ family
■ friends
■ neighbors
■ co-workers
■ people from church

Now let's broaden that a bit more:

■ Check with your doctor and local hospitals to see if there's a local support group. You can also call or check the Web sites of the major headache and Migraine organizations for listings of support groups.
■ Ask your doctor if he or she knows of another headache or Migraine sufferer who could use a "buddy." The doctor or someone on staff could call that person (or even more than one) and give the person your phone number. It certainly

couldn't hurt to have someone to talk to who has shared similar experiences.

∎ For emotional support and sharing information, there are great online resources. There are forums and groups/mailing lists with members who are very compassionate and supportive. Check the appendix for listings.

There will be times when we simply don't feel like running out to get cards and do other things that go along with being a "good friend." That can be tough on relationships and thus tough on our support systems. Some advance planning can work wonders in this department. Consider buying all your birthday cards the first of the year. You can address them and have them ready to mail in advance. Hallmark makes some great organizers for cards that allow you to mark dates to send them. Or just get an extra calendar and put each month's cards between the appropriate pages. You can leave them unsealed until it's time to mail them so you can add an appropriate last minute note. Don't wait for occasions to buy gifts. When you're out and see something you'd like to give someone as a gift, go ahead and buy it. Take it home and wrap it when you're feeling well. Put it in a bag with a note indicating what it is. When the occasion arrives, you'll be ready, whether you're feeling well or not. Buy your Christmas and holiday cards as soon as they come out for the season or even after the season the previous year. If you send many, consider using clear computer labels with a nice font for addressing the envelopes. Again, address them as soon as you buy them so they'll be ready. Your friends and family will be impressed that you always remember and manage to handle cards and gifts so well even when you're not. This is great reinforcement and thanks for the people who form your support system.

If the people who form your support system have done things for you such as fixing meals, watching your children, running errands, and so forth, sometime when you're feeling well, offer to return the favor. It will help alleviate the feelings of being a burden that most of us have from time to time, and it will make people feel truly appreciated.

Sometime around Thanksgiving, consider a special giving of thanks for those who make up your support system. This can take just about any form, depending on how much you're able to do. For example:

- If your headaches and Migraines are well enough controlled to allow you to plan a gathering at your home or an outing, plan a special Thanksgiving with those who support you. Depending on your family situation, combining this with the traditional Thanksgiving holiday may work, but remember— your family needs to be made to feel ultraspecial. Thus, combining the two events may or may not be a good idea.
- If you have a special talent for making something special, consider pacing yourself through the year to make a small gift for each person in your support system. Then give them at Thanksgiving time with a personal note.
- As you feel up to it, sit down with some nice stationery and write a personal thank-you note to each person and mail or deliver them near Thanksgiving.

It doesn't really matter much what it is you do. What matters is making the effort to let each of these people know you're thankful they're a part of your life.

Now I'm going to get all touchy-feely on you. Life is just too short. There are no guarantees of who will or won't still be here tomorrow. We're living with Migraine disease and/or headaches. We all live with the basic uncertainties that go with life—traffic accidents, sudden illnesses, and other events that take people from us unexpectedly. I'm not being gloomy, just realistic, when I say we never know how much longer anyone we know will be with us. I certainly didn't think my father would die at the age of fifty-nine.

That's only nine years older than I am now. So you know what? When you love someone, you should tell that person. Never miss a chance to tell someone. Apply that to the people in your support system, too. I can guarantee you that the people who offer you the most support do so because they love you.

Our Internal Support System

Just as we can't expect our doctors to do all the work to help us gain control over our Migraines and headaches, we need to look to ourselves for part of our own support. Yes, I realize that sounds strange. "Support system" seems to imply external forces, not ourselves. Not so. Everything starts and ends with us. Everyone else supplies input along the way. The best support system in the world can't help us emotionally if we're not in the proper mode to receive support. If we've already made up our minds to be in a doom-and-gloom mood, everyone else's best efforts will fail. In psychology, this principle is known as the "self-fulfilling prophecy." If you expect the worst, that's what you'll get. If you leave the door open for success, it's more likely to happen. Starting to make sense now? In chapter 19, we'll talk about keeping ourselves going. I've also made a few little reminders we can keep around to bolster our spirits. They're available online, too, where you can print them in color or black and white. Just go to www.HelpForHeadaches.com/lwfiles/reminders.htm.

Summary

Building a support system is vital. There are many sources of support, some obvious, some not so obvious. Be willing to think creatively about sources of support. It can be surprising where we find the support we need. Beyond building our support system, we have to remember to appreciate those who are a part of that system and let them know we appreciate them.

Bookmarks for some of the reading you're going to do:

Knowledge IS Power!

Learning about headaches will help me gain control over them and be more in control of my life.

I WILL Prevail!

**For you, from:
Teri Robert
HelpForHeadaches.com**

Knowledge IS Power!

Learning about Migraine disease will help me gain control over it and be more in control of my life.

I WILL Prevail!

**For you, from:
Teri Robert
HelpForHeadaches.com**

19

Empowerment over Headaches and Migraines

What do I mean when I say "empowerment over headaches and Migraines"? I mean our becoming empowered and taking back or retaining control of our lives . . . not letting headaches or Migraine take over. We've already discussed many elements of empowerment:

- Awareness: As those around us and the general public become more aware of headache disorders and Migraine disease, we'll have more support.
- Knowledge: As we learn more, we have more power, more control.
- A good medical team, including the right doctor: A good medical team means fewer worries for us. It also means a good source of knowledge.
- A strong support system: A good support system can take away a great deal of the isolation and loneliness that goes hand in hand with chronic illnesses. It can also provide you with a safety net and allow you to occasionally let yourself be cared for without feeling guilty.

Now I want to talk about another element that leads to empowerment. Whatever our beliefs, it's essential that we keep the spiritual and emotional parts of ourselves healthy, too. Part of our empowerment comes from within us and/or, depending upon our beliefs, from God or a higher power. For purposes of this discussion, I'll use the word *god* with a lowercase "g" to indicate whatever higher power each of us holds dear. It's impossible to overestimate the power of prayer and faith. That power can sometimes compensate for a great many inadequacies in other places. If we picture our empowerment as a brick wall, our prayer, faith, and inner strength are the mortar that holds it all together and completes it, making it whole and strong.

Prayer and faith help us remember we're not alone. They can tie a knot in the end of our rope when we're nearing the end. They help us see a small miracle and smile when we need it most. Prayer and faith remind us that whatever happens, god does not leave us. We can't understand the reasons for pain and illness, yet we know our faith will help us persevere.

Whatever your beliefs, please remember to take time to nurture your spiritual side. When you're concerned about illness, pain, doctors, and medications, it's easy to neglect taking that time. Don't. It's more important now than ever. One of the strongest recommendations I can make to each of you—whether you believe in god or not—is to take at least thirty minutes each and every day just for yourself. Even if you have children and a job, you can find thirty minutes a day for yourself. If you're a spiritual person, you may want to spend it in prayer and meditation. Remember to spend a few minutes in thanksgiving each day. It's amazing the things you'll think of, and it will really give you a lift. Some people like to keep a daily journal of thanks. They discover that the exercise of finding at least one thing for which they're thankful every day, and writing it down, is very therapeutic. They can also turn to that journal in times of distress. If you're not a spiritual person, spend your "me time" taking stock of your emotional and mental state and making sure you're doing well. Spend that thirty minutes concentrating on yourself and centering and focusing yourself for the next twenty-four hours.

If you find yourself not coping well, don't be ashamed or embarrassed to seek help. Some headache and Migraine clinics have psychologists and psychiatrists on staff. It's not because anyone thinks the head pain their patients are experiencing is psychological. It's generally for two reasons:

1. Migraine disease and clinical depression are often comorbid (existing simultaneously with and usually independently of another medical condition) diseases. A psychological evaluation to see if we're experiencing clinical depression—and if we are, that we're being appropriately treated—is not only appropriate, it's excellent.
2. Chronic illnesses require special coping skills. An evaluation is often performed to see if we possess the coping skills we need so that we can be helped if we don't.

Sometimes it takes more courage to ask for help than it does to "suffer in silence." Please don't do that to yourself. If you're feeling depressed, it could be a medical issue as well as an issue of coping skills. Help is available on both counts. We owe it to ourselves to get that help if we need it. We owe it not only to ourselves, but to everyone who cares about us.

Some people with headaches and Migraine disease find that writing is very therapeutic. Some write just for themselves; some share their writing with others. Writing as therapy can take any form:

▪ a journal or diary where you express your feelings, vent them onto paper
▪ short stories

- poetry
- a combination of any or all types of writing

Here are a few poems written by headache and Migraine sufferers:

Migrainous Horror

by Becky

Waiting for Daddy to come home to rescue them,
the helpless three- and five-year-old children
watch their Mommy,
standing beside her silently, trying to be quiet nurses,
as she vomits and shakes permanent scary memories
into their young minds . . .
this fear created would go away . . .
if someone would smash my head

The embarrassing eye twitch and immediate plea
for dark and quiet,
the begging for items to decrease the flashes of light
and jaw pain would stop . . .
if someone would smash my head

The glasses would not hurt to wear and
having to "just function" through life for another chapter
would not happen . . .
if someone would just smash my head

Upon the tormenting Migrainous occasions,
the family and friends around you
would not think of the desperation and humiliation
that accompanies my sheer presence
as I walk into a room straight legged and stiff,

teeth clenched, searching for relief, a purse,
medication, cold rags, something to stop the nausea,
anything—
ANYTHING—to stop the throbbing, stabbing pain
when I KNOW that my head may explode at any moment,
the thoughts and feelings would go away . . .
   if someone would smash my head

The twitching, begging, guilt from instilling fear,
embarrassment, humiliation, flashing, shaking,
nausea, sleeping, drugging, ER visiting, helplessness,
searching, pain and more pain.
The horrific life consuming, life stealing, life altering,
life limiting Migraines would end . . .
   if someone would PLEASE smash my head

Asea
by Lisa Staley

Drowning in electric seas, I drift
Where naught I may do but surrender to the ebb
And flow—awaiting the inevitable swell.

I drift, gently awash in the tide,
Feeling the build of the current, the rise
Of sheer power—a fury fast approaching.

Against the rage of the undertow, the glistening
Shimmer of a million shattered droplets
Assault me—the roar cuts fast and deep

In breaking waves of pain.

MIGRAINE MILESTONES
by Dorrie Philbeck

With the onset of puberty I first complained,
these terrible headaches kept me detained,
with each monthly PMS curse also came
the commencement of this horrid migraine.

Our family physician did quickly proclaim,
"It's your sinuses that are to blame."
He immediately sought to "cure" my pain,
"Just take these sinus pills," he explained.

This treatment my mother sought to maintain,
wringing her hands, trying to hide her disdain,
she brought cold washcloths to lay over my brain.
Clearly, this therapy could not long sustain,
I was soon taking aspirin like sugarcane
trying to get rid of this frightful migraine.

Thus began the long search for a cure,
each new phase I learned to endure,
Treatments continued to prove more obscure,
but in counting my blessings I felt more secure.

Suffering today under this icepack
my throbbing head giving me no slack,
feeling the next moment my head's going to crack
Oh, how long do I have to endure this attack?!?

Then my dear granddaughter sits down by my bed
offering sweet prayers for my aching head,

she's often seen Papa with me bow his head,
"Bring healing and comfort, Lord," he's many times said.

The Lord gives me strength to get through this pain,
His promises help me feel whole again,
love will sustain me, that's why I proclaim,
"This inhumane migraine will not win the game!"

Empowerment over headaches and Migraine disease! If our headaches or Migraines are controlling our lives, we can take back that control. If they're not controlling our lives, we can make sure they don't. Keep these elements of empowerment in mind:

- awareness
- knowledge
- a good medical team, including the right doctor
- a strong support system
- staying strong mentally and spiritually

This is no more than what we deserve in life. Let's make sure we achieve it!

20

Advocacy Issues: Knowing and Claiming Your Rights

As if all the medical issues aren't enough, there are times those of us with headaches and Migraine disease find situations where we feel we aren't treated fairly. There's a good reason for that. We *aren't* always treated fairly. One of the reasons is that we have invisible illnesses. We can feel our pain, but there are no *visible* signs of these illnesses . . . no shaved heads from brain surgery, no casts from broken bones, nothing that other people can see. Let's take a look at some of the most common issues we face and what we can do.

Insurance Companies Limiting Doses of Triptans per Month

I list this one first because it's the one about which I get the most complaints. I offer you a real case as an example: A woman in Florida contacted me because she was having trouble getting her prescription for Maxalt filled. She and her doctor hadn't been successful in finding effective preventives yet, so he'd written her prescription for twenty-four Maxalt tablets. When she went to the pharmacy to pick it up, she was told her insurance company had limited that medication to twelve tablets. She called the insurance company but got no results. She called me; I called the insurance company. As I anticipated, the customer service representative (CSR) told me it was "because of FDA regulations." *Ha!* I told you I anticipated that one. I had called the FDA before calling the insurance company, and I was able to tell him that an FDA official had just told me the FDA has no jurisdiction over any insurance company. The FDA regulates the pharmaceutical industry, not the insurance industry, and no FDA regulations would have any effect on payment for prescription medications. The rather flustered CSR asked me for the name and phone number of the FDA official and asked if he could put me on hold. He came back on the line approximately fifteen minutes later with a different reason not to cover the Maxalt. He said that their medical review staff had "been told by experts that triptans are addictive." Offering to provide him with the names of excellent Migraine experts, I explained to him that triptans are not addictive and that the FDA-approved prescribing information even states very clearly that they're not addictive. He told me he'd have to consult their medical review staff and get back to me. In our next conversation, the CSR suddenly had a section of the patient's insurance policy to quote me. It stated that the plan had limits on certain medications, including Maxalt. Ahhh. Now if that were in her policy, it would make things totally different. I just happened to have a copy of her policy on my desk. It was one hundred pages long, so I asked him to please tell me what page that clause was on and we'd be able to close the case. Strange, but he couldn't tell me what page it was on. Someone had just given him the clause itself, not pointed it out in the context of her policy. At that point, I explained to the CSR that I would be publishing an article regarding the case on my About.com Web site in four days. The company was welcome to e-mail or fax me any comments they cared to make, and he was welcome to call me back to resolve the case.

Nothing happened. I published my article with the facts to that point. The day the article was published, the CSR phoned me asking where to find the article. I told him, and he was not happy. I told him that the headline and content of my article for the following week would depend totally upon what his company did with the case that week. He told me a staff pharmacist would contact me during the week to discuss it. Once again I issued an invitation for company officials to comment for my article. The week went by with no further contact, so I published an article summarizing events and stating that they still had not resolved the case. Just after the second article appeared, the patient was contacted by the insurance company and told the whole situation had been "an error." They not only started filling her prescriptions as written, but reimbursed her for the Maxalt she had paid for when she ran out of what they had covered.

In several other cases where I've contacted insurance companies on behalf of patients, their first response has also been "FDA regulations." Once that's shot down, those companies have blamed the limitations on a "review panel." When I offer my opinion that the patient's attending physician has expressed his orders in writing in the form of a prescription, and changing it by limiting the amount dispensed is practicing medicine without a license, they've been quick to tell me they have doctors on their review panels. My logical response is that those doctors could be brought up on charges of malpractice, since they've never reviewed the patient's medical records, let alone examined the patient. Interestingly enough, in approximately 75 percent of cases, that logic is followed by the insurance companies' reversing their decisions and removing their limits.

These are not isolated or unusual cases. Over one thousand Migraineurs and cluster headache sufferers have filed formal com-

plaints with me through my About.com Web site. If you find yourself in this situation, please don't just put up with it. Until we all
start standing up on this issue, it will continue. Call your insurance
company officials and do all you can to get them to reverse their decision. If your insurance is through your employer, talk to someone
in personnel or employee benefits about it. There are times when
such limitations are the result of the type of coverage purchased.

Being Viewed as a "Drug Seeker" When Seeking Treatment

Sigh. This is an unconscionable situation, and it arises all too often.
It happens most often in emergency rooms, but some people report
it happening in doctors' offices also. This is something else we have
to fight, and fight hard, and passionately, and to the end. I'm going
to give you a case example here that will show you why I feel so
strongly about this issue:

> CASE EXAMPLE: *Janice (name changed) had been commu-
> nicating with me via e-mail and telephone for a few months.
> She and her fiancé, James (name changed), had moved into
> their new apartment but placed their wedding on hold until
> her Migraines were better controlled, so they could enjoy the
> event. Janice was a thirty-two-year-old elementary school
> teacher who wanted two children of her own. James is a
> thirty-six-year-old architect. He'd have agreed to a house full
> of children if that was what Janice wanted, but he thought her
> plans of a boy and girl were perfect. Janice was doing every-
> thing "right." She was seeing a neurologist, taking preven-
> tives, using triptans as soon as a Migraine attack began, using
> rescue medications sparingly when triptans failed. She was
> keeping a perfect diary, had done an elimination diet, and*

had identified a few food triggers that she avoided faithfully. Her other triggers were fairly well identified, but not as easily managed. Weather changes and the fluorescent lighting in her classroom were two of her worst triggers. Since she'd been making no progress with her current neurologist, she was waiting for an appointment with a Migraine specialist. Even so, about once a month, a Migraine would spiral out of control, and James would need to take her to the emergency room.

James is what I'd call a model partner. When he learned Janice had Migraine disease, he told her he wanted to know more about it so he could help her. He was determined to understand the disease and be as helpful and supportive as humanly possible. We had also talked on the phone a couple of times.

More than once, Janice had expressed to me what many Migraineurs do—the frustration of being treated like a "drug seeker" in the ER. Although she'd been treated with suspicion and disrespect, by the end of each visit she had been able to convince someone to call her doctor, and the visit was resolved with her Migraine being treated appropriately.

Unfortunately, there came that horrible morning when I got a phone call from James. Janice had committed suicide the night before while he slept. She'd had a Migraine that required a trip to the ER. They immediately encountered a problem when, because he was not her spouse and did not have a medical power of attorney, he wasn't allowed to accompany her to the exam room. They decided not to push the point for fear of seeming "difficult." James told me he was "shocked beyond words when she came back out in less than half an hour." She told James that a doctor she'd never seen before had treated her. He'd come into the exam room, checked her reflexes, and *told the nurse what kind of injection to give her. Janice told him another doctor there had tried that before and it hadn't worked, and she asked him to call her doctor. The ER doctor replied, "I'm not calling anyone. I know how to treat people like you." By that time, the nurse was back and gave her the injection. Both the doctor and nurse left. The nurse returned with Janice's discharge papers. When Janice objected to being discharged because she felt no better, the nurse left, and the doctor returned. He told her to "vacate that bed for people who really need it" or he'd call security.*

After they got home, Janice and James went to bed. Janice got up and went into the bathroom. James heard water running into the bathtub and thought Janice was going to soak in a nice hot bath—something she often did when she had a Migraine. He drifted off to sleep waiting for her. In the morning, he awoke and instantly knew something was wrong. Janice was not in bed. He found her still in the bath, where she'd had a couple of glasses of wine, then cut her wrists. He called 911, but the bathwater and Janice were both cold already. It was too late.

As he told me what had transpired, James sobbed out of grief, anger, and guilt. Obviously, he was grieving at losing Janice. He was also angry, but he was not entirely certain with whom he should be angry.

James isn't alone in his anger. After I'd spoken with him, I beat the daylights out of my desk with a dictionary. My cats ran for cover! With whom should we be angry? I can think of several candidates:

▌ Obviously, the doctor who *mis*treated Janice in the emergency room.

▌ The ER nurse who could have tried to help Janice.

▌ What about the real "drug seekers" who go to ERs and fake pain to get opioids?

▌ Perhaps the Drug Enforcement Administration? There are times when it seems they'd rather persecute legitimate patients and doctors than enforce the laws on the books and go after the people who are selling and buying prescription drugs on the streets.

▌ Then there are politicians. The National Pain Care Policy Act of 2003 is still sitting in committee in the House of Representatives. At this rate, it may never make it to the floor for a vote. Does anyone remember how many politicians used passing a "Patient's Bill of Rights" as a campaign issue in 2000? Gee, where is it?

Most important, James is *not* to blame. That's difficult for him to remember. Our system is seriously dysfunctional and needs to be fixed, but I certainly don't know how it's going to happen. In the meantime, I suggest we all prepare the emergency care forms from chapter 14 and hope we don't have to go to the ER.

If you receive inadequate care in the ER, I urge you *not* to let it go. You may need to just go home that day, but that doesn't have to be the end of it. Stop and think. When your vital signs were checked, did whoever checked them ask you to assess your pain on a scale of 1 to 10? If not, the hospital was in violation of the standards set by the Joint Commission on Accreditation of Healthcare Organizations (JCAHO). JCAHO accreditation is necessary for a hospital to be eligible to bill Medicare, so that's important to them. Get a notepad, make note of that, and go on from there to make notes of what problems occurred during your ER visit. Then call the hospital administrator's office and request a face-to-face meeting with the hospital administrator and the person in charge of the emergency department. Type up your notes. Review them, and be sure they're as factual as possible without being overly emotional. Avoid confrontational wording. Make copies for everyone who will be at the meeting. If possible, take someone with you for support. If someone was with you in the ER, they're the ideal person to take to the meeting. Approach the meeting with a constructive attitude, and you'll be more likely to accomplish something. Rather than flat-out saying you think the ER is staffed with insufferable jerks, suggest that perhaps some education about headaches and Migraine disease would help avoid such unfortunate incidents. If you weren't asked to assess your pain, tactfully let them know that you're aware of the JCAHO standard and they didn't meet it. You can even say that you don't want to cause trouble for the hospital, so you're not going to report it to the JCAHO—this time.

If you can do this, you're trying to make things better not only for the next time you may have to go to the ER, but for every patient who walks through those doors. There are times when we must advocate for ourselves. If we let these things go, they'll never get better. Go for it!

Fighting Migraine Disease

When I reported Janice's suicide, many of my online readers were strongly impacted. Members of the Yahoo! group Migraine were so moved that they felt impelled to *do* something, something major. They came up with the idea of awareness wristbands for Migraine disease. The cost of the wristbands was generously underwritten by the GelStat Corporation, and the wristbands are available for the cost of shipping and the request of a small donation to a NGD nonprofit Migraine organization. Please visit its Web site at www. fightingmigrainedisease.com.

Have You Had Trouble Regarding Your Medical Records?

Copies of Our Medical Records

Over the last couple of years, we've all been having to sign more and more privacy notices when going for medical care. Have you noticed? That's because of HIPAA, the Health Insurance Portability and Accountability Act of 1996. Although the act originated in 1996, certain provisions didn't go into effect until later because of the time needed to make changes to records systems and procedures.

The last time I "fired" a doctor, I asked his receptionist for a copy of my records. She told me they couldn't be released to me, but the office would gladly send a copy to my new doctor. Wrong answer! Not only can those records be released to us, but doctors are required—by law—to do so, and to do so within thirty days unless you are given a good reason. Period.

Are There Errors or Something You Disagree with in Your Records?

We can ask to change any wrong information in our file or add information to our file if it is incomplete. For example, if we and our hospital agree that our file has the wrong result for a test, the hospital must change it. Even if the hospital believes the test result is correct, we still have the right to have our disagreement noted in our file. In most cases, the file should be changed within sixty days, but the hospital can take an extra thirty days if we are given a reason.

Preexisting Conditions

When changing from one insurance plan to another or getting medical insurance for the first time, medical conditions we already have are referred to as "preexisting conditions." They can make insurance more costly, or there can be an initial period during which treatment for that condition isn't covered. HIPAA sets regulations about how preexisting conditions must be handled by insurance companies, which makes getting or changing insurance plans easier and more equitable.

More Information About HIPAA from the U.S. Department of Health and Human Services

Who Must Follow HIPAA?

■ Most doctors, nurses, pharmacies, hospitals, clinics, nursing homes, and many other health care providers.

■ Health insurance companies, HMOs, and most employers.

■ Certain government programs that pay for health care, such as Medicare and Medicaid.

What Information Is Protected?

■ Information your doctors, nurses, and other health care providers put in your medical record.

■ Conversations your doctor has about your care or treatment with nurses and others.

■ Information about you in your health insurer's computer system.

■ Billing information about you at your clinic.

■ Most other health information about you held by those who must follow this law.

The Law Gives You Rights over Your Health Information

Providers and health insurers who are required to follow this law must comply with your right to:

■ ask to see and get a copy of your health records.

■ have corrections added to your health information.

■ receive a notice that tells you how your health information may be used and shared.

▮ decide if you want to give your permission before your health information can be used or shared for certain purposes, such as for marketing.

▮ get a report on when and why your health information was shared for certain purposes.

If you believe your rights are being denied or your health information isn't being protected, you can file a complaint with your provider or health insurer or file a complaint with the U.S. government.

The Law Sets Rules and Limits on Who Can Look at and Receive Your Information

To make sure that your information is protected in a way that does not interfere with your health care, your information can be used and shared:

▮ for your treatment and care coordination.

▮ to pay doctors and hospitals for your health care and help run their businesses.

▮ with your family, relatives, friends, or others you identify who are involved with your health care or your health care bills, unless you object.

▮ to make sure doctors give good care and nursing homes are clean and safe.

▮ to protect the public's health, such as by reporting when the flu is in your area.

▮ to make required reports to the police, such as reporting gunshot wounds.

Your Health Information Cannot Be Used or Shared Without Your Written Permission Unless This Law Allows It

For example, without your authorization, your provider generally cannot:

■ give your information to your employer.

■ use or share your information for marketing or advertising purposes.

■ share private notes about your mental health counseling sessions.

There's far more to HIPAA; it's quite extensive. For more information, contact the U.S. Department of Health and Human Services Office for Civil Rights toll-free at 1-866-627-7748 or visit its Web site at www.hhs.gov/ocr/hipaa.

Are You Uninsured and Having Problems Affording Medications?

Almost all of the pharmaceutical companies have patient assistance programs that provide medications at no charge for patients who have no prescription insurance coverage and meet income guidelines. The income guidelines are more generous than you might think, so these programs are worth checking into. They do require paperwork to be completed by your doctor. Usually they send a three-month supply of the medication to your doctor's office for you. If your need still exists, you can reapply before you run out. For a directory of patient assistance programs, see www.HelpFor Headaches.com/lwfiles/rx-assistance.htm.

Is Missing Work Causing You Problems?

This can be a real problem for people with chronic headaches or Migraines. Hopefully your employer will be willing to work out something with you. A letter from your doctor may be helpful if you're missing many workdays.

If the company you work for employs fifty or more people, check out the Family and Medical Leave Act. Covered employers must grant an eligible employee up to a total of twelve work weeks of unpaid leave during any twelve-month period for one or more of the following reasons:

■ For the birth and care of the newborn child of the employee.

■ For placement with the employee of a son or daughter for adoption or foster care.

■ To care for an immediate family member (spouse, child, or parent) with a serious health condition.

■ To take medical leave when the employee is unable to work because of a serious health condition.

You can get more information about FMLA from your local office of the U.S. Department of Labor or online at www.dol.gov/esa/whd/fmla/. If you're not covered by FMLA, talking to the Department of Labor will still help by giving you information on any other laws that may be applicable to you.

Are You Disabled by Your Headaches or Migraines?

You may qualify for Social Security Disability Insurance (SSDI) or Supplemental Security Income (SSI). SSDI and SSI are the largest of several federal programs that provide assistance to people with disabilities. While these two programs are different in many ways, both are administered by the Social Security Administration (SSA), and only individuals who have a disability and meet medical criteria may qualify for benefits under either program.

SSDI is financed with Social Security taxes paid by workers, employers, and self-employed persons. To be eligible for a Social Security benefit, the worker must earn sufficient credits based on taxable work. Disability benefits are payable to disabled workers, disabled widow(er)s, or adults disabled since childhood who are otherwise eligible. Auxiliary benefits may be payable to a worker's dependents as well. The monthly disability benefit payment is based on the Social Security earnings record of the insured worker on whose Social Security number the disability claim is filed.

SSI is financed through general tax revenues. SSI disability benefits are payable to adults or children who are disabled or blind, who have limited income and resources, who meet the living arrangement requirements, and who are otherwise eligible. The monthly payment varies up to the maximum federal benefit rate, which is standardized in all states, but not everyone gets the same amount because it may be supplemented by the state or decreased by other countable income and resources.

When you apply for either program, the SSA collects medical and other information from you and makes a decision about whether or not you meet Social Security's definition of disability.

The definition of disability under Social Security is different from that under other programs. Social Security pays only for total disability. No benefits are payable for partial disability or for short-term disability.

Disability under Social Security is based on your inability to work. You are considered disabled under Social Security rules if you cannot do work that you did before and the SSA officials considering your case decide that you cannot adjust to other work because of your medical condition(s). Your disability must also last or be expected to last for at least one year or to result in death.

This is a strict definition of disability. Social Security program rules assume that working families have access to other resources to provide support during periods of short-term disabilities, including workers' compensation, insurance, savings, and investments.

To determine if you are disabled, the SSA uses a series of five steps:

1. **Are you working?**

   If you are working in the current year and your earnings average more than $810 a month, you generally cannot be considered disabled. If you are not working, the SSA will go to Step 2.

2. **Is your condition "severe"?**

   Your condition must interfere with basic work-related activities for your claim to be considered. If it does not, the SSA will find that you are not disabled. If your condition does interfere with basic work-related activities, the SSA goes to Step 3.

3. **Is your condition found in the list of disabling conditions?**

   For each of the major body systems, the SSA maintains a list of medical conditions that are so severe, they automatically mean you are disabled. If your condition is not on the list, the SSA has to decide if it is of equal severity to a medical condition that is on the list. If it is, the SSA will find that you are disabled. If it is not, the SSA goes to Step 4.

4. **Can you do the work you did previously?**

   If your condition is severe but not at the same or equal level of severity as a medical condition on the list, then the SSA must determine if it interferes with your ability to do the work you did previously. If it does not, your claim will be denied. If it does, the SSA proceeds to Step 5.

5. **Can you do any other type of work?**

   If you cannot do the work you did in the past, the SSA will see if you are able to adjust to other work. It considers your medical conditions and your age, education, past work experience, and any transferable skills you may have.

If you cannot adjust to other work, your claim will be approved. If you can adjust to other work, your claim will be denied.

You can get more information or apply for either SSDI or SSI at your local SSA office. SSDI applications are taken online at s3abaca.ssa.gov/pro/isba3/wwwrmain.shtml and by telephone at 1-800-772-1213. SSI applications are not taken online but are taken by telephone at 1-800-772-1213. Another helpful Web link is the Disability Starter Kit at www.ssa.gov/disability/disability_starter_kits.htm.

Be prepared. Almost all SSDI and SSI applications are denied the first time, and an appeal is necessary. On the positive side, we're seeing more people approved for Migraine and chronic headaches than were approved before. If your application is denied, you may want to hire an attorney for your appeal. There are many attorneys who will take such cases on a contingency basis. They get paid only if your appeal is successful. Then they get a percentage of the lump sum that's paid retroactively from the time you're declared to have been disabled. When you get to this point, your attorney might find it helpful to see copies of some favorable disability case decisions. You can find four of them on the site of MAGNUM, the National Migraine Association, at www.migraines.org/disability/disablgl.htm.

There are many advocacy issues that affect those of us with headaches and Migraine disease. When you think about it, all of the pain treatment advocacy issues affect us, too. That's one reason I joined the American Pain Society and a reason I belong to several advocacy groups. Would you like to help change things? There are many opportunities for advocacy that don't involve huge commitments. There are plenty of times when writing a couple of letters can be a big help. If you're interested, check www.HelpForHeadaches.com/lwfiles/advocacy.htm and the appendix of this book. In the appendix, you'll find a listing of advocacy groups. On the Web site, you'll always be able to find those listings *plus* current advocacy projects that could use a bit of your time and assistance.

PART FOUR

What Does It All Mean?

21

If Your Situation Seems Hopeless

If you retain two thoughts from this book, let them be these two:

1. You are *not* alone.
2. There *is* hope.

Much of this has been said elsewhere in this book, but it's important enough to bring it all together and repeat it here. If your situation seems hopeless, tie a knot in the end of your rope, find some support to help you along your journey, and start looking for a good headache and Migraine specialist to work with you.

Five years ago, I thought I was doomed to spending more than half of my life in bed, debilitated by Migraines, never able to plan anything. Now I have one treatable Migraine about every six or eight weeks. I've seen people with daily Migraines who are now down to a couple of manageable Migraines a month. There are people I've worked with who had chronic daily headaches that kept them from being able to work, play with their kids, or have a social life. With education, good treatment, and a solid support system, they are now controlling their headaches instead of having their headaches control them.

Rather than telling you about the success stories I've heard and read, let me share a few with you.

Success Story #1

I saw my neuro today. Great lady, but dang, I wish I were as skinny as she is . . . no, wait, if I were, I'd not be able to handle my motorcycle. :)

Okay . . . she has told me I don't need to see her for a year unless something drastically changes like the Topamax stops working or the clusters (God forbid!) start up again. She is very pleased with the progress I've made since I've started back on Topamax and said she's using me for her poster child this week. :)

Success Story #2: Making Reachable Goals, Then Reaching Farther

I have never posted under successes because I feel like every time I celebrate, it soon ends. But I will be brave. Up until last week, I had my longest stretch major Migraine episode free since the beginning of symptoms . . . twenty-five days. Yes, I was so so excited, but instead of that being good enough, I am always waiting for thirty days; that is my goal. Instead of being bummed about missing thirty, I will take your advice and celebrate the twenty-five! I believe the cycle was broken by my new medicine, a bad choice for me, as I had daily episodes for five days and then threw up the white flag and stopped the med.

Now for celebration number two. Today I am Migraine-

*free. The best part of that? I had a hot date with my two
teenage sons for Valentine's Day and was able to enjoy every
minute of it.* Woo-hoo!!

SUCCESS STORY #3

*I am soooo happy, I can't stand it. I was in a car accident in
November of 1998, and since then have had the chronic daily
headaches, Migraines that put me out for the count for days
twice a week, and doctor after doctor who told me that it
couldn't be related to the car accident, that wasn't "how it
worked." I had had Migraines before that, but only one every
month or two, nothing like the agony I was dealing with after
the accident.*

*Well, I found a wonderful neuro that said, Let's eliminate
the medicine possibilities, then go on from there. After seven
months of switching meds every two to four months, she admitted that we had done enough to convince the insurance
that we had done what we could. She sent me to a pain specialist. He agreed that there was no way my Migraines should
happen the way they have been. The first visit he tried a treatment even he doubted the efficacy of, but it was what the insurance had agreed to. He had me come back a few weeks
later for the first occipital nerve block. Afterwards, I went for
nine days pain-free.*

*When I came back, he said that was better than he had
hoped and that he would do another treatment, and I
wouldn't have to come back until the Migraines started to
bother me again. I was scared to death, sure that I would be
back in three weeks.*

*It has been a month and a half. I have had two slight Mi-
graines, both treated with Relpax and went away within a
couple of hours.*

Success Story #4: I Saved the Most Dramatic for Last!

Dear Teri,

I just had to write to you to thank you for all you help. To thank you for all the times you encouraged me, gave me pep talks, listened while I cried, and even gently scolded when I was ready to give up. How is it that I was ready to give up on myself, but you wouldn't give up on a stranger? Anyhow, I had to let you know that you were right about firing my doctor's "sorry butt" and hiring a "real doctor." It caught me off guard the first time you said that, but now it's funny. True, but funny. When I was able to get an appointment with your doctor, I still didn't really believe it could make so much difference. After all those years with a headache or Migraine every day, it was too much to believe in. You know? But things there were just as you described them. The doctors and nurses really listened to me for a change.

It would have been easy to get discouraged at first because the first preventive medicines made me sick and didn't help anyway. But I remembered what you said, and the nurse and the doctor were super encouraging. They reminded me that we were just getting started, and there were still lots of things to try.

To get to the present, it's been a year now, and I've accepted that my Migraines are a disease that I'll always have. The good part is that I only get one or two Migraines most months, and that's such a huge improvement that it's almost as good as a cure. Imitrex didn't do much for me, but Maxalt works great.

Teri, I have a life again! Now I know that when my husband left because of my Migraines, he actually did me a favor. I met a guy who takes me to dinner or a movie now and then.

It may get serious, or not, but I have a life. Thank you so much for never giving up on me.

Although it may not seem like it sometimes, there has been an astonishing amount of progress made in headache and Migraine disease treatment over the last ten years, and it's continuing! Effective preventive regimens can be found for 95–98 percent of people with Migraine disease and headache disorders. A good specialist can also offer hope for the few people who don't fall into that vast majority. They can work with those patients to establish pain management regimens that allow them to at least have some pain-free time, even if it's not possible to make all their time pain-free.

If a doctor tells you there's nothing more that can be done for you, don't believe it for a second! You just stand right up to that doctor, tell him he's an undereducated wimp and his sorry butt is *so* fired! Then go home and have yourself a good cry to release the tension, if you need to, and find yourself a good specialist. I promise you there are excellent doctors out there who will not give up on you as long as you don't give up on them or yourself.

22

Summary and Review

It's impossible to review all the main points of the book here, but we can start with these:

▮ Optimal health care can be achieved only when patients are educated about their health and patients and physicians work together as treatment partners in an atmosphere of mutual respect.

▮ Headache and Migraine management should consist of six parts:

1. *Education.*

2. *Trigger identification and management: identifying what brings on your headaches or Migraine attacks and learning how to manage those triggers.*

3. *A good preventive regimen.*

4. *Appropriate abortives (medications that actually stop a Migraine attack rather than just masking the pain).*

5. *An emergency plan and pain management for times when abortives fail.*

6. *A strong support system.*

▐ Tension-type headaches are the most common, affecting at least 80 percent of us sometime in our lives. At this point in time, that's 187 million Americans.

▐ Migraines are not headaches. Migraine is a genetic neurological disease affecting nearly 33 million Americans. A headache may be one symptom of a Migraine attack.

▐ Although rare, Migraine attacks can cause strokes, which can kill. Don't take chances. If your symptoms are dramatically different from or more severe than those you're used to, get help.

▐ Cluster headaches are possibly the most severely painful of all head pain. They affect more men than women.

▐ We must be in charge of our health care team. If our doctor doesn't listen to us, won't answer questions, or doesn't give the same respect he or she expects to receive, we need to fire his or her sorry butt and move on! Our doctors work for us.

▐ It may be necessary to seek the care of a true headache and Migraine specialist to get the care we need.

▐ An orgasm can trigger an exertional headache or a Migraine attack *or* it can abort a Migraine attack. It all depends on the individual.

▐ There are five elements to *empowerment* over headaches and Migraine:
  1. *Awareness.*
  2. *Knowledge.*
  3. *A good medical team, including the right doctor.*
  4. *A strong support system.*
  5. *Staying strong mentally and spiritually.*

▐ A strong support system is as important as good medical care.

▐ None of us is alone with our illness. We have quite a lot of fine company in one another.

▐ There is a great deal of hope for good treatment.

Have you been hard on this book? Did you mark it up as you read it? Whatever your habits are as you read a book, I hope you found what you needed here. Actually, this book wasn't finished. It can never be finished because there is new information coming out so quickly. My Web site for this book, www.HelpForHeadaches. com, is a permanent site. There you will be able to find new information as it becomes available. I invite you to visit the site, subscribe to my free e-mail newsletter, join our discussion forum, and participate in our live online chats. For me, running the site and interacting with others who have headaches and Migraine disease is part of "Living Well" with this disease. There's a sense of family that develops as we spend time conversing, even online, with others who share our experiences. I wish each of you success in your treatment and the best possible support system. If you'd like to contact me, you're welcome to do so through my Web site.

23

My Personal Approach to My Headaches and Migraines

It needs to be emphasized that this is my personal approach to my own headaches and Migraines. It has been developed over more than three years of treatment with a top Migraine specialist, and I have never added an element to my regimen without first discussing it with him. I'm glad to share my approach with you. Doing so may give you some insights and thoughts to discuss with your own doctors.

My approach to my health is holistic. That means I believe in addressing all parts of myself—physical, emotional, intellectual, social, and spiritual. Why? Let me explain to you why I take this approach. It's my belief that all of those aspects make a complete person. Unless all of them are as well as possible, I will not be as well as possible. The emotional, intellectual, social, and spiritual aspects also affect my physical health. In fact, each aspect affects the others; they're intertwined. Why should I "settle" for addressing only part of my health and feeling somewhat better when I can feel far better by addressing all aspects of my health? I deserve and owe it to myself to be as well as possible in all regards. I could spend thousands of dollars on Migraine treatment, but if I don't address the other aspects of myself, I'm cheating myself out of being as well as I can be, being all I can be to my family and friends, and accomplishing all I can accomplish with my life. It's not as complicated as it sounds, and you don't have to be a "fanatic" (as some of you may be thinking) to live this way.

Physical

Caring for the physical aspect of myself is more than just going to the doctor and taking my medications. That's part of it, of course, and I'll get to that. When I began treatment with my specialist, the frequency and severity of my Migraines had caused me to become a pretty sedentary person. At least that was a good excuse. The truth was that I could have done more to work some physical movement into my days, but I didn't. Although Dr. Young didn't really push me, he did encourage me to be as physically active as I was able to be. He reminded me that even a little bit of physical activity helps, and it doesn't necessarily have to be "exercising"; there's activity in everyday life. I began by doing a series of stretching exercises every single day, sometimes more than once a day. It's a series of stretches I learned when I took a fencing class for physical education in college. They gently stretch the entire body, and I found I could do them unless in the midst of a severe Migraine.

As the frequency of my Migraines has decreased, I've felt more like being active and have done so. I'll be honest: I'm not the type of person who is going to go outside and walk or participate in sports when the temperatures are extreme or when it's raining. It's just not going to happen. On the other hand, a treadmill in my home office, with a television in front of it, is a different matter. That I will do. You don't have to walk for long periods of time for it to be beneficial. Good thing, too! When I started using the treadmill, five minutes was about all I could manage, so I'd use it several times a day. Before long, the length of time I could walk comfortably on the treadmill increased. With an interesting television show or some good music to go with it, the time flies, and I get a good cardiovascular workout! Since I've been diagnosed with coronary artery disease, exercise has become an even higher priority to me. I've kept up with my stretches and the treadmill, and I've added Pilates. I tried yoga but quickly decided it was designed to kill me. Pilates is very gentle but effective, and there are a number of good videos and DVDs if you don't want to go out and take classes.

Another issue was nutrition and what I was drinking throughout the day. Again, another disease plays a role. I have type 2 diabetes, so it's important that I watch what I eat to keep my blood sugar levels controlled. Diet sodas and other diet drinks were what I drank most of the time. Water? Never. That changed when I learned that caffeine can make drinks less effective for keeping the body hydrated. Also, since I wanted to lose weight, I knew I needed to drink water. Now I drink about a gallon of iced water every day.

Over the course of my treatment, Dr. Young and I worked through medications and dietary supplements to find a regimen that would reduce the frequency and severity of my Migraine attacks as much as possible. There's no cure for Migraine disease, but to me, having up to two months pain-free between Migraine attacks is the next best thing. Dr. Young worked with me carefully so that we didn't increase the number of medications I take any more than necessary. I was already taking medications for high blood pressure and clinical depression. Since medications for those conditions are often excellent for Migraine prevention, he changed my meds to different ones that were more likely to address both depression and Migraine prevention. He also discovered that I have a condition known as pseudotumor cerebri. It causes my body to produce too much cerebrospinal fluid, which causes the fluid pressure to be high and was triggering some of my Migraines. We had to add a medication to treat that and one additional medication when I developed chronic daily tension headaches on top of the Migraine disease. Ultimately, when my successful regimen was set, we had added two prescription medications and three dietary supplements. There are days when I feel like a walking pharmacy and want to pitch all my meds, but I will not give up the progress I've made. If the price is taking these medications for the rest of my life, so be it.

Emotional

With the complexities of today's society, it's hard enough to be emotionally healthy when we're well. When we have a debilitating illness or disease, it becomes even more difficult. It's important that we be aware of our emotions and pay attention to them. Negative emotions, if not dealt with, can spiral out of control all too quickly. In my case, I have to deal with clinical depression. About ten years ago, I found myself in a period of time where I simply couldn't shake my feelings of depression and hopelessness, even though everything in my life was going well. I'd find myself sitting in the middle of the floor crying for no reason. Watch a sad movie? Forget it! That's when I began medical treatment for clinical depression, which is a disease. I've since learned that there's a link between that disease and Migraine disease. I take stock of how I'm feeling emotionally on a regular basis. If it doesn't match my circumstances, I know I need to address it. Relaxation exercises can also be extremely helpful for emotional health. At Dr. Young's recommendation, even though my Migraines and headaches are well controlled now, I listen to my favorite relaxation CD every day.

Intellectual

We all need to be intellectually stimulated. It keeps us sharp and alert. It also keeps me from getting horribly bored. Reading, studying, and learning continue to be a regular part of my life. We live in an amazing time for learning. With a proliferation of books, great magazines, plus the wealth of good content on the Internet, we have more opportunities for learning than at any time in history. With the Internet, we can even read newspapers from all over the world. Amazing!

Social

Mankind is a social creature. We aren't meant to live solitary lives. There is medical evidence that people who have strong friendships are healthier. Supportive and positive friendships can increase our hope when dealing with illness and trauma. Increased hope is associated with higher levels of immune system functioning. I'm sure many of you can relate to this—when my Migraines were at their worst, many of my friendships seemed to disintegrate. That made me fully realize the value and depth of the friendships that survived. Keeping in touch with friends was essential when my Migraines were at their worst because I felt so isolated. It's also part of my ongoing headache and Migraine treatment because it keeps me healthier.

Spiritual

When I say "spiritual," I don't necessarily mean religious, although that can be part of it. The spirit is the very essence of who we are, and it needs nurturing and nourishing. I believe in God, so prayer is part of nourishing my spirit. That won't be the case for everyone. Whether you believe in God, a god of a particular faith, Mother Earth, or another higher being, communicating with that entity or entities is part of caring for your spirit. That's not all of it, though.

It's another of my beliefs that we can't give our best in any relationship with another person unless we truly like and love ourselves. I used to have a terrible temper and a reputation for that temper. I realized I don't like people with terrible tempers, and that meant there was part of myself I didn't like. Over a period of several years, I worked hard to build patience and other ways of handling situations in which I'd have normally displayed that temper. Now, most people don't think of me as a person with a bad temper at all. My point is that we can work to become the kind of person we want to be, to have the kind of spirit we want. For me, that means frequent prayer and meditation to achieve a peaceful and calm spirit.

Some Extra Help Along the Way

There are some complementary therapies that I employ on a regular basis for physical, emotional, and spiritual health:

- ▮ *Aromatherapy:* Earlier in this book, I discussed aromatherapy as a complementary treatment for headaches and Migraine. Aromatherapy is also a valuable tool for emotional and spiritual health. I often use essential oils in a diffuser to release them into the air around me. Incense is another form of aromatherapy I employ. By choosing different oils and incense, I can address my needs at any particular time. As I wrote this book, I often used one or the other to increase concentration and creativity or to help me relax. I also continue to use them to help relieve the nausea of Migraines and help me relax during an attack.
- ▮ *Crystal therapy:* Another complementary therapy discussed earlier in this book, crystal therapy can be used for a variety of reasons and in a variety of methods. I use crystals to

aid with relaxation, concentration, and reduction of headaches and Migraines.

- *Meditation:* Meditation is a tool I find very helpful during a
  headache or Migraine. It's what often gets me through until
  my medications take effect. It helps me remain calmer and
  fight the panic that tends to strike me during an especially
  bad Migraine attack. I also use meditation on a daily basis
  for spiritual health.

Please Do This for Yourself

There is a great deal we can do for ourselves to fight headaches and
Migraine disease. Hopefully, by the time you've read this far, you realize that there's far more we can do than you realized. We're not
powerless. I began a daily routine a couple of years ago that I have
continued and will continue for the rest of my life. In my opinion, it
would be beneficial for everyone, even the healthiest of people. Try
setting aside thirty minutes of "me time" every day. Take the phone
off the hook. Turn off the television. Shut yourself in a room by
yourself. If you're traveling and sharing a hotel room or are in another similar situation, explain your need for thirty minutes of silence. What you do with that thirty minutes is up to you. You may
need to experiment a bit to find the best use of that time, and it may
not always be the same. I generally light a candle or some incense
and spend that thirty minutes in prayer and meditation. You may
find it a good time to write in a journal or do other things for yourself. Just be sure it's quiet time for yourself.

Summary

It's been a long trip from my first Migraine at the age of six through years of horrid Migraines to today, when they're well controlled. One of the most valuable things I've learned is that successful treatment is made up of many parts. It will vary for each of us, and it will take searching—and perhaps some failures along the way—to meet with success. If you're not there yet, keep going. It's well, very well, worth it.

24

As you can imagine, my e-mail is often filled with questions. Two years ago, Dr. John Claude Krusz (see his bio in appendix E), a highly qualified specialist, offered to help me answer questions for an "Ask the Clinician" feature on my About.com Web site. Between the two of us, we've published the answers to hundreds of questions in addition to all the questions I answer via e-mail. We cannot diagnose or give medical advice online, but we can educate and offer information. Here are some of the questions we receive most often:

Q: Is it possible to have a Migraine without having a headache?

A: *Absolutely. A Migraine actually consists of up to four phases. Not all Migraineurs experience all phases, and an individual's Migraine attacks can vary. Migraine attacks without the headache are often described as "silent" or "acephalgic" Migraines.*

Q: Help! I've started getting a severe headache when I reach orgasm. What is it, and what can I do?

A: *You need to see your doctor to have these headaches diagnosed. They may be coital headaches, which are a form of exertional headache. If so, your doctor can probably recommend a medication to take before sexual activity to prevent the headaches.*

Q. Are there preventive medications for cluster headaches?

A. *Yes. The same medications that are used as preventives for Migraine are often helpful preventives for cluster headaches.*

Q. Are there diagnostic tests to confirm that you have Migraine disease?

A. *Unfortunately, no. Doctors diagnose Migraine disease by reviewing the patient's personal and family medical history and their symptoms, performing a neurological examination, and ruling out other causes for their symptoms.*

Q. My doctor recommended a hysterectomy to reduce my Migraines. Is this a good idea?

A. *Absolutely not. There is no way to predict the outcome. Your Migraines might decrease, but they might also increase or stay the same. If that's your doctor's best advice, find a new doctor.*

Q. I just turned fifty, and my doctor says I'm too old for triptans. Is this true?

A. *No. Whether or not triptan therapy is appropriate should be determined by the state of the patient's health, not his or her age. Some doctors stop prescribing triptans for patients over fifty because the risk of cardiovascular disease increases with* *age. It's not unreasonable for doctors to request a cardiovascular workup if we're going to continue with triptan therapy past that age, but most doctors will continue prescribing triptans if the workup shows no problems.*

Q. What "Migraine diet" can I follow to help prevent Migraines?
A. *There is no one diet because we all react so differently to foods. Each of us needs to do an elimination diet to determine what, if any, foods are Migraine triggers for us. In an elimination diet, we cut out all the common potential trigger foods, then add them back into our diet one at a time. That lets us know if one of them is a trigger for us.*

Q. I've had the worst headache of my life for the last two days. What should I do?
A. *Whenever our symptoms change, we should let our doctors know. When we're experiencing the worst headache of our life, especially one lasting so long, we need to call our doctor or go to the emergency room to be sure it is a headache or a Migraine attack and not something else.*

Q. Can Migraines cause thinning hair?
A. *There is no clinical evidence of Migraine causing hair to thin. If you're taking medications, it may be a side effect of one or more of them. Check with your doctor or pharmacist about the potential side effects of your medications.*

Q. Will my Migraines decrease or go away after menopause?
A. *Unfortunately, only time will tell. For some women, the frequency of their Migraines does decrease after menopause. For a few, it increases. For yet others, there's no change at all. Anecdotally, it seems that women whose primary Migraine*

trigger is their menstrual cycle are more likely to experience a decrease in Migraine activity after menopause than women whose Migraine patterns aren't affected by their cycles.

Q. Should I be worried about the increased stroke risk caused by having Migraines?

A. *Unless you're at high risk for stroke otherwise, not really. We should all be aware that Migraine disease increases our stroke risk and talk to our doctors about a healthy lifestyle to decrease stroke risk, but even with Migraine disease, the risk is still very small. The average stroke prevalence in women in the general population is 9 per 100,000, which represents absolute risk. If women with Migraines have an average of 2.16 times greater risk, that's about 20 per 100,000, still a very low absolute risk. On oral contraceptives, the absolute risk is about 75 per 100,000. Thus, I'd say "aware" is a better word than "worried."*

Q. How long is a "fair trial" of a preventive medication?

A. *It depends somewhat on the type of medication, but it can take up to three months to give a preventive medication a fair trial and know if it's going to work.*

Q. I've tried everything for headache prevention. What can I do now?

A. *First of all, don't lose hope. Unless you're about 110 years old, it's virtually impossible for you to have tried everything for prevention. There are so many possible preventives, not to mention the nearly endless combinations of preventives, that you couldn't possibly have tried them all. It is possible that you've tried all of them your current doctor knows. That's when it's time to move on to a true headache and Migraine specialist. Since they treat only head pain patients, they have* *far more experience. They also get more ongoing training in the field. It's truly amazing the difference a good specialist can make in our treatment.*

Q. My daughter's Migraines never seem to go away. She wakes up with a throbbing headache daily, feels nauseated, is sensitive to light, motion, and sound. Her latest doctor said she does not have Migraines because "Migraines go away." Is it possible to have daily or nearly daily Migraines?

A. *Unfortunately, yes, it is possible to have daily or nearly daily Migraines. As for your daughter's doctor, fire his sorry butt and find someone who knows more about Migraine disease. This doctor is not going to be able to help your daughter with that way of thinking.*

Q. Can a transient ischemic attack (TIA) be mistaken for a Migraine? Is there any type of Migraine that can present itself with similar symptoms—that is, drooping mouth, weakness down one side of the body, and double vision?

A. *Yes, a TIA can be mistaken for a Migraine and vice versa, as the symptoms are very similar. Again, yes. There are a couple of forms of Migraine that can present these symptoms. It is very important that you see your doctor and get a correct diagnosis. These forms of Migraine require extra precautions and different treatment from that for "regular" Migraines. If your doctor can't pinpoint it, you may need to seek care from a Migraine specialist.*

Q. Have there been any studies about the effects of marijuana on Migraines?

A. *The literature on the effect of marijuana on Migraines is very poor. As you can imagine, it is not a topic the government will support readily. Most "studies" are anecdotes, and formal re-*

search is lacking. There is some theoretical information why cannabinoids may be useful in treating Migraines and pain, and there are also small published studies suggesting that marijuana can increase headaches. It's an interesting topic that needs study.

Q. Once a person develops analgesic rebound (from taking too much pain medicine in the first place or whatever), can that person ever again, sometime in the future, be able to take pain medicine with normal results?

A. *In general, if the offending medications causing the rebound have been removed for enough time, it should be possible to use pain medications judiciously (infrequently) if needed. The larger picture is that, hopefully, better categories of medications will have been found to treat ongoing Migraines so that the older medications don't need to be used.*

Q. Is it unusual to have a tender spot on my head on the side where my Migraines occur?

A. *No. You should be sure to mention this to your doctor, but sore spots on the scalp, either during or after a Migraine, are a common occurrence with Migraineurs.*

Q. Are Migraines hereditary?

A. *Yes. Migraine is now known to be a genetic neurological disease. Some Migraineurs don't think there's a family history but, upon closer examination, realize there actually is. It's possible that, in previous generations, your relatives' Migraines were referred to as "sick headaches," were mistaken for sinus headaches, or were mild and infrequent enough that they weren't really noticed much.*

Q. What's the probability that I'll pass on Migraine disease to my children?

A. *If one parent has Migraine disease or a family history of it, there's a 50 percent chance that children will inherit the disease. If both parents have Migraine disease or a family history, there's a 75 percent chance that children will inherit the disease.*

Q. How long should I tolerate side effects of a preventive medication before calling my doctor?

A. *That depends a great deal upon the medication and the type of side effect. Try to remember to ask your doctor that question when he or she prescribes a new medication. When you pick up your prescription at the pharmacy, read and keep the patient information sheet so you can refer to it later if you need to. Some side effects such as slight drowsiness or nausea will often subside as the body adjusts to the medication. However, some medications in use as preventives have potentially serious and permanent side effects, such as vision problems. So if there are any questions about side effects, it's always best to call the doctor and be sure and safe.*

Q. Do tension headaches start across the forehead or in the back of the neck?

A. *It depends on the person. The pain of a tension headache can start either place.*

Q. Is there a cure for Migraine disease?

A. *Not at this time. In my opinion, if one is to be found, it will lie in the genetic research that's being done on Migraine disease, but it's still a long way off. I think the genetic research will lead to more effective preventives first.*

Q. Can a person have more than one type of headache disorder?

A. *Absolutely. That's not at all unusual. For example, I have both tension-type headaches and Migraine disease. Some people have both Migraine disease and cluster headaches. Choose the combination, and it can happen.*

Q. Why does my face hurt when I have a Migraine?

A. *A Migraine attack affects the trigeminal nerve, which has three branches. One goes around the eye, one to the upper jaw area, the third to the lower jaw area. Impulses sent to the trigeminal never can cause your face to hurt during a Migraine attack.*

Q. Is it unreasonable to expect my doctor to stick around long enough to answer my questions when I have an appointment?

A. *No, it's not. However, doctors are more receptive when we use our appointment time as efficiently as possible. One of the best things you can do is make up a list of your questions in advance of your appointment and give a copy of it to your doctor at the beginning of your appointment. That way, he or she already knows you have questions and can pace the appointment to have time to answer them.*

Q. How can I tell the difference between a Migraine and a headache?

A. *There are several differences:*

- *The type of pain differs. Headache pain is usually a steady ache. Migraine pain is usually a throbbing pain that often seems to throb with your pulse (pulsatile).*
- *The location of the pain. Migraine pain is most often, although not always, unilateral (on one side). Headache pain is more likely to be bilateral (both sides).*

▌ *The pain of a Migraine is made worse by activity such as bending over, climbing stairs, and so on. Headache pain generally is not.*

▌ *A headache is usually not accompanied by nausea, vomiting, sensitivity to sound, or sensitivity to light.*

Q. Which is better for a headache or migraine—a cold pack or hot pack?

A. *In both a headache and a Migraine attack, neither is better than the other. It depends on personal preference. I even know one person who uses both. She puts a hot pack on the back of her neck and a cold pack on her forehead.*

Q. Why have antiseizure drugs become so popular for Migraine prevention?

A. *For one thing, they're working well for many people. Also, it's thought that the root cause of Migraines is related to overactive neurons in the brains of Migraineurs. Another name for antiseizure medications is neuronal stabilizing agents. They essentially calm neurons. The current theory is that they help prevent Migraine attacks by this mechanism.*

Q. Why do I crave salt after a severe Migraine?

A. *You may well become dehydrated as part of your Migraine, especially if you have a lot of nausea or vomiting. This could easily account for salt craving.*

APPENDIX A: GLOSSARY

Medical Terms

Abdominal Migraine: A form of Migraine most commonly seen in children. The main symptoms are nausea, vomiting, and abdominal pain, but no headache phase. Children who have abdominal Migraines tend to develop Migraine with or without aura as adults.

Abortive Medications: Medications used to "abort" a Migraine attack or cluster headache. These medications are not pain relievers. They work in the brain to stop the attack at its sources.

Acupressure: The application of pressure or localized massage to specific sites on the body to control symptoms such as pain or nausea. Also used to stop bleeding.

Acupuncture: The technique of inserting thin needles through the skin at specific points on the body to control pain and other symptoms.

Acustimulation: Mild electrical stimulation of acupuncture points to control symptoms such as nausea and vomiting.

Acute: Of short duration, rapid and abbreviated in onset, in reference to a disease. Acute is a measure of the time scale of a disease and is in contrast with "subacute" and "chronic." "Subacute" indicates longer duration or less rapid change. "Chronic" indicates indefinite duration or virtually no change.

Adjunctive Therapy: Treatment that is given in addition to the main treatment to make it work better.

Adverse Reaction/Adverse Event: An unwanted side effect of treatment, aka side effect.

Agonist: A drug that shows an affinity for and stimulates a receptor.

Allodynia: Sensitivity to touch that would otherwise be pleasant or non-painful.

Analgesic: A medication that relieves pain.

Analgesic Rebound Headache: Headache caused by medication overuse. Characterized by continuous dull head pain throughout the day with periods of increased pain. The general recommendation for avoiding rebound is not to use medications from the same class more than two or three days per week.

Aneurysm: A localized widening of an artery, vein, or the heart, typically a bulge where the wall is weakened and may rupture.

Anorexia: Suppression of appetite.

Antidepressants: A family of medications used to prevent or treat depression. The antidepressant drugs include selective serotonin reuptake inhibitors (SSRIs), monoamine oxidase inhibitors (MAOIs), tricyclic antidepressants, tetracyclic antidepressants, and others.

Antiemetics: Medications used to prevent or treat nausea and/or vomiting.

Anti-Inflammatory: An agent, such as a medication, intended to reduce inflammation and the associated pain and stiffness.

Aphasia: Loss or impairment of the power to use or comprehend words. Aphasia can be a symptom of a stroke, Migraine attack, brain injury, or other conditions.

Ataxia: Incoordination and unsteadiness due to the brain's failure to regulate the body's posture and regulate the strength and direction of limb movements. Ataxia may be a consequence of disease in the brain. It can also be a symptom of a Migraine attack or stroke.

Aura: The second of four phases of a Migraine attack. Only approximately 25 percent of Migraineurs experience aura. The symptoms may include:

■ visual: flashing lights, spots in vision, zigzag lines, blurry vision, temporary loss of vision
■ smell: olfactory hallucinations—smelling odors that aren't actually present
■ auditory: auditory hallucinations—hearing sounds that aren't actually there
■ aphasia: difficulty thinking of words and/or speaking
■ hypersensitivity to touch and feel
■ vertigo (sensation of moving around in space)
■ tingling of the face and/or extremities

Barbiturate: Medications that are derivatives of barbituric acid used especially as sedatives, hypnotics, and antispasmodics.

Basilar-Type Migraine (previously called basilar artery Migraine or basilar Migraine): Migraine with aura symptoms clearly originating from the brain stem and/or from both hemispheres simultaneously affected, but no motor weakness.

Bilateral: Occurring on both sides.

Biofeedback: The technique of making unconscious or involuntary bodily processes (as heartbeat, respirations, or brain waves) perceptible to the senses in order to manipulate them by conscious mental control.

Calcium Channel Blockers: A class of medications originally developed to treat hypertension. They're now used for additional purposes, including prevention of headaches and Migraine attacks. Calcium channel blockers inhibit the movement of calcium into the muscle cells of the heart and arteries. Calcium is needed for these muscles to contract. Thus, calcium channel blockers lower blood pressure by decreasing the force of the heart's pumping action and relaxing the muscle walls of the arteries.

Cataract: An opacity of the lens of the eye. Cataracts generally form as a result of aging, trauma, endocrine or metabolic disease, or intraocular disease or as a side effect of the use of tobacco or certain medications.

Central Nervous System: The brain and spinal cord.

Cerebrospinal Fluid (CSF): Fluid that surrounds and fills in the spaces around the brain and spinal cord.

Chi: In Asian medicine, the blockage of energy flow through the twelve meridians.

Chronic: Long-term or lasting.

Chronic Daily Headache (CDH): Headache occurring daily or almost daily, at least fifteen days per month.

Chronic Paroxysmal Hemicrania (CPH): A rare syndrome that presents as multiple, short, severe headaches that occur daily. CPH differs from cluster headaches in that the headaches are shorter (one to two minutes each), much more frequent (averaging fourteen times a day), and strike women more than men. CPH responds nearly 100 percent of the time to treatment with indomethacin.

Cluster Headaches: Series of headaches, typically occurring in men, that are intense, recurring, felt near one eye, and often associated with nasal congestion, rhinorrhea, and watering of the affected eye.

Comorbid: Existing simultaneously with and usually independently of another medical condition.

Conjunctival Injection: The forcing of a fluid into the conjunctiva, the mucous membrane that lines the eyelids.

Daily Headache: Headache occurring daily or nearly daily—at least twenty out of thirty days.

Diplopia: Double vision; seeing two images of an object at the same time.

Dysarthria: Impairments or clumsiness in the speaking of words due to diseases that affect the oral, lingual, or pharyngeal muscles. The patient's speech may be difficult to understand, but there is no evidence of aphasia.

Dysphasia: Impairment of speech.

Edema: Local or generalized condition in which the body tissues contain an excessive amount of tissue fluid. Although many people think of edema as occurring only in the extremities, such as legs and ankles, it can occur in most body tissues.

Embolus: A mass of undissolved matter present in a blood or lymphatic vessel and brought there by the blood or lymph. Example: blood clot.

Endorphins: Chemicals manufactured in the brain, spinal cord, and many other parts of the body. They are released in response to neurotransmitters and bind to certain neuron receptors (the same ones that bind opiate medications). Endorphins act to suppress pain and produce a calming effect. They are often called "the body's own painkillers."

Episodic: An event that is distinctive and separate although part of a larger series. Many diseases are episodic in nature with symptom-free periods punctuated by episodes of the disease in full force.

Extraocular: Outside the eye, as in extraocular eye muscles.

Familial Hemiplegic Migraine: Migraine with aura including motor weakness and at least one first- or second-degree relative has Migraine with aura including motor weakness.

Feverfew: An herb sometimes used in the prevention of Migraine. Not regulated by the FDA. Anecdotally known to help, but there have been no controlled studies to date.

Gene: The fundamental unit of DNA that controls inherited characteristics, including some diseases.

Hemicrania Continua: Persistent unilateral (one-sided) headache. It is usually unremitting, but there have been reports of rare cases of remission. Hemicrania continua is responsive to the medication in-domethacin.

Hormone Replacement Therapy (HRT): Use of supplemental hormones, usually conjugated estrogen and progestin, to treat hormonal deficiency states; relieve menopausal vasomotor symptoms; and manage post-menopausal atrophic vaginitis.

Hypacusia: Impaired hearing.

Hypertension: Greater than normal tension or tone. Usually used to indicate blood pressure higher than the "normal" range of 120/80.

Ice Cream Headache: Severe pain in the palate caused by eating ice cream or other similarly cold foods too quickly.

Idiopathic: Without clear pathogenesis or without recognizable cause, as of spontaneous origin.

Intractable Migraine: Sustained, severe Migraine and accompanying symptoms that are not effectively terminated by standard outpatient intervention. May evolve to a chronic and continuing form, similar to chronic daily headache.

Ipsilateral: Occurring on the same side as another symptom.

Ischemic Stroke: A stroke due to diminished blood supply to the brain or a particular area of the brain (for instance, the lodging of an embolus from the heart in an artery of the brain).

Lacrimation: The secretion and discharge of tears; tearing.

Macular Degeneration: Loss of pigmentation in the macular region (the region that provides central vision) of the retina. It usually affects people over fifty and is a common disease of unknown etiology that produces central visual field loss. It is the leading cause of permanent visual impairment in the United States.

Magnetic Resonance Angiography (MRA): Diagnostic radiography that uses the characteristic behavior of protons (and other atomic nuclei) when placed in powerful magnetic fields to make images of the blood vessels.

Magnetic Resonance Imaging (MRI): Diagnostic radiography that uses the characteristic behavior of protons (and other atomic nuclei) when placed in powerful magnetic fields to make images of tissues and organs.

Medulla Oblongata: The lowest part of the brain stem, continuous with the spinal cord above the level of the foramen magnum of the occipital bone.

Meningismus: Symptoms of meningitis without the actual illness and accompanying inflammation.

Menstrual Migraine: Migraine triggered by the hormonal fluctuations of a woman's menstrual cycle.

Migraine with Aura: Formerly called "classic Migraine," a genetic neurological disease manifesting in attacks of reversible focal neurological symptoms that usually develop gradually over five to twenty minutes and last less than sixty minutes; the full attack generally lasts four to seventy-two hours. Headache with the features of Migraine without aura usually follows the aura. Less common, the headache lacks Migrainous features or is totally absent.

Migraine Without Aura: Formerly called "common Migraine," a genetic neurological disease manifesting in attacks lasting four to seventy-two hours. Typical symptoms of the head pain are unilateral (one-sided) location, pulsating quality, moderate to severe intensity, worsening by physical activity, and nausea and/or photophobia and phonophobia.

Migraineur: A person who has Migraine disease.

Migrainous Infarction/Migrainous Stroke: One or more Migrainous aura symptoms associated with an ischemic brain lesion in appropriate territory demonstrated by neuroimaging.

Miosis: Abnormal contraction of the pupils, possibly due to irritation of the oculomotor system or paralysis of the dilators.

Monocular: Occurring in one eye.

Monosodium Glutamate (MSG): Chemical additive found in seasonings or Chinese food. MSG may sometimes trigger Migraine attacks in susceptible individuals.

Neurologist: Doctor specializing in diagnosis and treatment of diseases of the nervous system.

Neuron: A nerve cell that has the ability to transmit and receive nervous impulses.

Neurotransmitters: Chemicals occurring naturally in the brain that transmit messages from one nerve cell to another. In discussing Migraine, the neurotransmitter we talk about most often is serotonin. Another involved in Migraine is norepinephrine.

Oculomotor: Relating to eye movements.

Orbit: The bony, pyramid-shaped cavity of the skull that contains and protects the eyeball.

Over-the-Counter Medications: Medications available without a prescription; aka OTC medications.

Pain: Sensation of discomfort, distress, or agony resulting from the stimulation of specialized nerve endings. It serves as a protective mechanism (induces the sufferer to remove or withdraw).

Pain Threshold: The least experience of pain that a subject can recognize. Pain is always the experience of the patient and is individual; the stimulus intensity is an outside event.

Pain Tolerance: The greatest level of pain that a patient is able to tolerate. Pain is a subjective experience, hence pain tolerance level is the subjective experience of the particular patient and has the same clinical limitations as the pain tolerance level.

Paresthesia: Abnormal or unpleasant sensation often described as numbness or as a prickly, stinging, or burning feeling.

Parasympathetic Nervous System: The craniosacral division of the autonomic nervous system.

Paroxysmal Dyskinesia: Repeated, sudden, involuntary movements.

Pericranial: Pertaining to the periosteum of the skull, the periosteum being the fibrous membrane that lines the skull.

Periumbilical: Around the naval.

Phonophobia: Increased sensitivity to sound.

Photophobia: Increased sensitivity to light.

Pons: A broad mass of chiefly transverse nerve fibers conspicuous on the ventral surface of the mammalian brain at the anterior end of the medulla oblongata.

Postdrome: The phase of a Migraine attack following the headache phase. During postdrome, a person may feel tired or "hung over."

Preventive Medication: Medication taken to prevent an illness or symptoms.

Prodrome: The first phase of a Migraine attack. Person may be irritable or unusually sensitive to light or noise and may notice some fluid retention. May last for one or two days or just a few hours before other phases begin.

Prophylactic Medication: Preventive medication.

Ptosis: Dropping or drooping of an organ or part, as the upper eyelid from paralysis.

Pulsatile: Pulsating; characterized by a rhythmic beat.

Receptor: A structure in the cell membrane that combines with a drug, hormone, infectious particle, or chemical mediator to alter the function of the cell.

Rhinorrhea: A thin, watery discharge from the nose.

Sacrum: The triangular bone situated dorsal and caudal from the two ilia between the fifth lumbar vertebra and the coccyx.

Scintillation: Perception of twinkling light of varying intensity that can occur during the migraine aura.

Scotoma: Area of decreased or lost vision.

Serotonin: A naturally occurring derivative of tryptophan. Found in the cells of the brain, in platelets, and in the intestine. In the central nervous system, it is a key neurotransmitter. In the blood vessels, it is released from platelets when blood vessel walls are damaged; aka 5-hydroxytryptamine.

Serotonin Receptor Agonist: Medication that attacks Migraine at its source by selectively binding to receptors in the brain that regulate the release of serotonin.

Status Migrainous (Migrainousus): Severe, unrelenting Migraine headache associated with nausea and vomiting that lasts longer than seventy-two hours, with less than four hours of relief while awake, and may not be manageable under outpatient care. Patients in status Migrainousus are at increased risk of Migrainous stroke.

Stroke: Sudden loss of neurological function caused by vascular injury to the brain.

Supraorbital: Located above the orbit.

Sympathetic Nervous System: The thoracolumbar division of the autonomic nervous system.

Synapse: The space between the junction of two neurons in a neural pathway.

Tension Headache: Pain is on both sides of the head, is pressing and steady, rather than pulsating, is usually mild and does not cause incapacity, and is not worsened by ordinary daily activities. There is no associated nausea or sensitivity to light and noise. (Definition from the International Headache Society.)

Thoracolumbar: Related to the thoracic and lumbar parts of the spinal cord; denoting their ganglia and the fibers of the sympathetic nervous system.

Tinnitus: Ringing, hissing, or buzzing sound in the ears.

Trigeminal Nerve: The trigeminal nerve functions both as the chief nerve of sensation for the face and the motor nerve controlling the muscles of mastication (chewing). It gets its name from having three branches or divisions. The ophthalmic division carries sensations to the area around the eye, the maxillary carries sensations to the area of the upper jaw, and the mandibular division carries sensations to the area of the lower jaw.

Trigger: Stimulus that in interaction with the body constitutes a physiological trigger that brings on a headache or Migraine attack.

Unilateral: Occurring on one side.

Vascular: Pertaining to the channels that carry body fluids, usually used in connection with the blood vessels.

Vasoactive: Affecting the dilation or constriction of blood vessels.

Vasomotor: Pertaining to the nerves that innervate the smooth muscle in the walls of arteries and veins and thereby alter or preserve vascular tone.

Vertigo: The sensation of moving around in space (subjective vertigo) or of having objects move about the person (objective vertigo).

Abbreviations

These abbreviations are medical abbreviations, abbreviations used in writing prescriptions, and abbreviations for various organizations. Although some aren't necessarily related to Migraine disease and headaches, they may come in handy.

AAC: American College of Cardiology

AACP: American Association of Colleges of Pharmacy

AAFP: American Academy of Family Physicians

AAMC: Association of American Medical Colleges

AARP: American Association of Retired Persons

abd: abdomen; abdominal

abx: antibiotic

a.c.: before meals

ACHE: American Council for Headache Education, American College of Healthcare Executives

ad lib: freely

AD: right ear

ADA: Americans With Disabilities Act, American Diabetes Association, American Dental Association

adj: adjust

ADL: activity of daily living

ADR: adverse drug reactions

ADS: alternative delivery system

aer: aerosol

AHA: American Hospital Association, American Heart Association

AHRQ: Agency for Healthcare Research and Quality

Alt: alternate or alternative

AMA: American Medical Association

amt: amount

ANDA: abbreviated new drug approval

antihist: antihistamine

antituss: antitussive

APAP: acetaminophen

APhA: American Pharmaceutical Association

APN: advanced practice nurse

applic: application

art: arterial

AS: left ear

ASA: aminosalicylic acid (aspirin)

AU: each ear

bib: drink

b.i.d.: twice daily

b.i.n.: twice nightly
BP: blood pressure
buc: buccal
BUN: blood urea nitrogen
bx: biopsy
BZD: benzodiazepine
C: cream
c: with
CA: cancer
CAD: coronary artery disease
cap: capsule
CAPD: continuous ambulatory peritoneal dialysis
CBC: complete blood count
cc: cubic centimeter
CCB: calcium channel blocker
CCU: coronary care unit
CDC: Centers for Disease Control
CDV: cardiovascular disease
CH: chewable
CHD: coronary heart disease
chemotx: chemotherapy
CHF: congestive heart failure
CL: total body clearance
Cmax: maximum concentration
CMP: complete metabolic panel
CNS: central nervous system
COB: coordination of benefits
COBRA: Consolidated Omnibus Budget Reconciliation Act
CON: certificate of need
conc: concentration
CPAP: continuous positive airway pressure
CPR: cardiopulmonary resuscitation, computerized patient record
CPT: current procedural terminology
CrCl: creatinine clearance
crm: cream
CSF: cerebrospinal fluid
CT: computerized tomography
CVA: cerebrovascular accident
d: day
daw: dispense as written, no substitutions

DBP: diastolic blood pressure (the lower of the two numbers)
D/C: discontinuation or discontinue
ddx: differential diagnosis
decong: decongestant
decr: decrease or decreased
defic: deficiency
div: divided
dl: deciliter
DOS: date of service
DPI: dry powder inhaler
ds: disease
Dx: diagnosis
dysfxn: dysfunction
dz: disease
ECG: electrocardiogram (same as EKG)
EEG: electroencephalogram
efferv: effervescent
EKG: electrocardiogram
elev: elevated
elix: elixir
EMG: electromyelogram
EMT: emergency medical technician
ENT: ear, nose, and throat specialist
ERT: estrogen replacement therapy
esoph: esophageal
ESRD: end stage renal disease
ETT: endotracheal tube
extr: extract
FA: folic acid or folate
FDA: Food and Drug Administration
FNP: family nurse practitioner
FP: family practitioner
freq: frequency
FUO: fever of unknown origin
fxn: function
G: gel
g: gram
GC: glucocorticoid
gel: gel or jelly
GERD: gastroesophageal reflux disease

GI: gastrointestinal

GP: general practitioner

gran: granules

gt: drop

GTT: glucose tolerance test

GU: genitourinary

h: hour

Hb: hemoglobin

HbA1c: glycosylated hemoglobin; blood test showing average blood glucose level for the previous ninety days

Hct: hematocrit

HCTZ: hydrochlorothiazide

HD: hemodialysis

HMO: health maintenance organization

HRT: hormone replacement therapy

h.s.: bedtime

ht: height

hx: history

hypersens: hypersensitivity

IA: into the artery

IBW: ideal body weight

ICU: intensive care unit

ID: intradermal

IHS: International Headache Society

IM: intramuscular

incr: increase or increased

IND: investigational new drug

infus: continuous infusion

INH: oral inhaler or orally inhaled

inj: injection or injectable

intraureth: intraurethral

intxn: interaction

IP: inpatient

IT: intrathecal

IU: international unit

IV: into the vein

IVP: intravenous pyelogram

JCAHO: Joint Commission on Accreditation of Healthcare Organizations

kg: kilogram

l: liter
L: lotion
LA: long acting
lb: pound
LCP: licensed clinical psychologist
liq: liquid
LOC: loss of consciousness
lot: lotion
loz: lozenge
LPN: licensed practical nurse
LR: lactated ringer's injection
LT: long-term
LTC: Long-term care
MAGNUM: National Migraine Association
malig: malignancy
MAO: monoamine oxidase
max: maximum
MC: mineralocorticoid
mcg: microgram
MDI: metered dose inhaler
mEq: milliequivalent
Mfr: manufacturer
mg: milligram
MI: myocardial infarction
min: minute
ml: milliliter
mm: millimeter
mmHg: millimeters of mercury
MMPI: Minnesota Multiphasic Personality Inventory
mo: month or month-old
mod: moderate
MRI: magnetic resonance imaging
MS: multiple sclerosis, master of science
msec: millisecond
MTF: military treatment facility
MTX: methotrexate
MVP: mitral valve prolapse
NAS: nasal inhaler or nasally inhaled
NDA: new drug approval
NDC: national drug code

NEB: nebulized inhalation

nec: necessary

ng: nanogram

NG: nasogastric

NHF: National Headache Foundation

NIAMS: National Institute of Arthritis and Musculoskeletal and Skin Diseases

NIH: National Institutes of Health

NINDS: National Institute of Neurological Disorders and Stroke

NL: normal

NLM: National Library of Medicine

non rep: do not repeat

noxt: at night

NP: nurse practitioner

NQWMI: non-Q wave MI

NS: not significant or normal saline

NSAID: nonsteroidal anti-inflammatory drug

NTE: not to exceed

N/V: nausea/vomiting

O: ointment

OA: osteoarthritis, open access

OC: oral contraceptive

OCP: oral contraceptive

O.D.: right eye

ODT: orally disintegrating tablet

oint: ointment

OP: outpatient

OPT: outpatient physical therapy

O.S.: left eye

OTC: over-the-counter

OTIC: instilled in the external ear canal

O.U.: each eye

oz: ounce

P: powder

PA: physician's assistant

PAD: peripheral artery disease

p.c.: after meals

PCI: percutaneous coronary intervention

PCN: penicillin

PCP: primary care physician

PE: pulmonary embolus
PET: positron emission tomography
pil: pill
pkg: package
pkt: packet
plt: platelet
p.o.: orally; by mouth
POS: point of service
postop: postoperatively
ppd: packs per day
PPO: preferred provider organization
p.r.: per (by) rectum
preop: preoperatively
prep: preparation
prev: previously
p.r.n.: as needed
prophyl: prophylaxis
pt: patient
pts: patients
PV: given vaginally or by vaginal suppository
PVB: premature ventricular beat
PVC: premature ventricular contraction
pwdr: powder
q.2h.: every two hours
q.3h.: every three hours
q.4h.: every four hours
q.6h.: every six hours
q.8h.: every eight hours
q.12h.: every twelve hours
q.ac: before every meal
q.am: every morning
q.d.: every day; once daily
q.h.: every hour
q.hs.: every evening
q.i.d.: four times per day
q.mo.: every month
q.noon: every noon
q.od.: every other day
QoL: quality of life
q.pc.: after every meal

q.pm: every afternoon/evening
q.q.h.: every four hours
q.s.: as much as is required
q.wk: every week
R: ringer's injection
RA: rheumatoid arthritis
RDA: Recommended Daily Allowance
resp: respiratory
R/O: rule out
Rx: prescription
rxn: reaction
S: solution
s.: without
SBP: systolic blood pressure (the top number)
SC: subcutaneous
sec: second
sev: severe
SH: shampoo
shmp: shampoo
s.l.: sublingual; under the tongue
SMX: sulfamethoxazole
SODLAC: sodium lactate, $1/6$ molar
sol: solution
solub: soluble
s.o.s.: if necessary
SR: sustained release
ss: half
stat: immediately
supp: suppository
suppl: supplement
susp: suspension
sx: signs or symptoms
syr: syrup
t$1/2$: half-life
tab: tablet
tbsp: tablespoon
t.d.s.: to be taken three times daily
TIA: transient ischemic attack
t.i.d.: three times a day
t.i.n.: three times a night

tinc: tincture
tmax: time to maximum concentration
TMP: trimethoprim
TOP: topical route
TPN: total parenteral nutrition
troc: troche
TSH: thyroid-stimulating hormone
tsp: teaspoon
tx: treatment or therapy
txp: transplant
U: unit
ung: ointment
URI: upper respiratory infection
US: ultrasound
ut. dict: as directed
UTI: urinary tract infection
vagC: vaginal cream
w/: with
WBC: white blood cell
WHA: World Headache Alliance
WHO: World Health Organization
w/in: within
wk: week
w/o: without
wt: weight
XR: extended release
XRTx: radiation therapy
y: year
yo: year old
yr: year

APPENDIX B: SUPPLEMENTAL MATERIALS AVAILABLE ONLINE FOR FREE REFERENCE AND/OR DOWNLOAD

Note: If you don't have Internet access at home, check your public library. Most libraries now have computers with Internet access that are available to the public.

Chapter 2

- Medical History Checklist: www.HelpForHeadaches.com/lwfiles/history-checklist.htm
- Headache/Migraine Diary: www.HelpForHeadaches.com/lwfiles/diaries.htm

Chapter 5

- List of Potential Migraine Trigger Foods: www.HelpForHeadaches.com/lwfiles/trigger-foods.htm
- Pathways of Migraine Illustration: www.HelpForHeadaches.com/lwfiles/pathways.htm

Chapter 10

- Directory of Recommended Headache and Migraine Specialists: www.HelpForHeadaches.com/lwfiles/specialists.htm
- Questions to Ask New Doctors: http://HelpForHeadaches.com/lwfiles/new-doc-questions.htm

Chapter 13

- Pathways of Migraine Illustration: www.HelpForHeadaches.com/lwfiles/pathways.htm

Chapter 14

▌ Forms to help get better ER care:
www.HelpForHeadaches.com/lwfiles/emergency-forms.htm

Chapter 17

▌ Letters to share with friends who don't understand:
www.HelpForHeadaches.com/lwfiles/letters.htm

Chapter 20

▌ Directory of pharmaceutical company Patient Assistance Programs: www.HelpForHeadaches.com/lwfiles/rx-assistance.htm
▌ Advocacy resources and opportunities:
www.HelpForHeadaches.com/lwfiles/advocacy.htm

APPENDIX C: RESOURCES

This Book's Web Site

For the latest information about headaches and Migraine disease, the forms and other materials in this book, a free e-mail newsletter, discussion forum, chat room, and more, please visit www.HelpForHeadaches. com.

Fighting Migraine Disease

When I reported Janice's suicide (see page 199), many of my online readers were strongly impacted. Members of the Yahoo! group Migraine were so moved that they felt impelled to *do* something, something major. They came up with the idea of awareness wristbands for Migraine disease. The cost of the wristbands was generously underwritten by the GelStat Corporation, and the wristbands are available for the cost of shipping and the request of a small donation to a NGD nonprofit migraine organization. Please visit its Web site at www. fightingmigrainedisease.com.

Information and Support

About Headaches and Migraine: www.headaches.about.com
Another of my Web sites, this site is a comprehensive source for information and support for Migraine disease and headaches. It includes articles and other information, a discussion forum, and an e-mail newsletter.

About Holistic Healing: www.healing.about.com

If you're interested in holistic healing, this is a great resource for articles and other information about all kinds of therapies—Reiki, aromatherapy, chakra balancing, crystal therapy, feng shui, and more.

About Alternative Medicine: www.altmedicine.about.com

This is a great site for information on all kinds of alternative therapies, including acupuncture, aromatherapy, biofeedback, massage therapy, reflexology, and more.

About Stress Management: www.stress.about.com

We can all use some help with day-to-day stress at times. This site is perfect for that or for anyone who needs more information. You'll find comprehensive articles and information, great stress management tips, a discussion forum, and a free e-mail newsletter.

All Info About Headaches and Migraine:
www.headaches.allinfoabout.com

This is another of my sites, similar to my other sites with articles, a forum, and a newsletter. The main difference is that this one also deals with forms of chronic pain other than head pain.

American Council for Headache Education (ACHE):
www.achenet.org

ACHE is a nonprofit, patient-oriented organization dedicated to empowering headache sufferers through education and supporting them by educating their families, employers, and the general public.

19 Mantua Road
Mt. Royal, NJ 08061
Phone: 856-423-0258

American Pain Foundation: http://www.painfoundation.org

The American Pain Foundation is an independent nonprofit organization serving people with pain through information, advocacy, and support. Their mission is to improve the quality of life of people with pain by raising public awareness, providing practical information, promoting research, and advocating to remove barriers and increase access to effective pain management.

201 N. Charles Street, Suite 710
Baltimore, MD 21201-4111

ClusterHeadaches.com: www.clusterheadaches.com
ClusterHeadaches.com is an online worldwide cluster headache support group.

Drugs.com Drug Information Online: www.drugs.com.
An excellent resource for information on medications. Also includes a pill identifier; look for the link at the bottom of any page of the site. It's a free site, but it is a for-profit site, so expect the typical banner and text ads.

HeadacheCareCenter: www.headachecare.com
Headache Care Center is a nationally recognized referral center for clinicians and patients seeking an interdisciplinary and personalized approach to the treatment of headache.

The Jefferson Headache Center:
www.jefferson.edu/headache/home/index.cfm
The Jefferson Headache Center is one of the leading headache centers in existence. Its Web site offers basic information about headaches and Migraine disease and some treatments as well as information about the clinic, its staff, and services.
8130 Gibbon Building
111 South 11th Street
Philadelphia, PA 19107
Phone: 215-955-2243

MAGNUM, the National Migraine Association: www.migraines.org
MAGNUM was created to bring public awareness using the electronic, print, and artistic mediums to the fact that Migraine is a true biologic neurological disease; to assist Migraine sufferers, their families, and co-workers; and to help improve the quality of life of Migraine sufferers worldwide. It is the only major nonprofit organization dedicated solely to Migraine disease and Migraineurs. Its site offers a wealth of information about the disease, treatment options, disability, legislation, and other vital matters.
113 S. St. Asaph Street
Alexandria, VA 22314
Phone: 703-739-9384

Migraine Crisis Line (MCL): www.migrainecrisisline.org

The MCL is a nonprofit organization created to meet the need for around-the-clock, seven-days-a-week support for Migraineurs and other head pain sufferers. Crisis line volunteers are sufferers themselves. Thus, callers can be assured of talking with someone who can relate to their situation. The MCL can help callers with basic information, finding doctors, prescription assistance programs, and moral support. They cannot, however, give medical advice and cannot take the place of callers' physicians.

Phone: 304-863-8404

The National Headache Foundation (NHF): www.headaches.org

The NHF is a nonprofit organization dedicated to educating headache sufferers and health care professionals about headache causes and treatments. As part of this effort, the NHF sponsors live support groups in cities across the United States. Its Web site offers articles, tip sheets, educational modules, and more.

820 N. Orleans, Suite 217
Chicago, IL 60610
Phone: 888-643-5552

The National Institute of Neurological Disorders and Stroke (NINDS): www.ninds.nih.gov

The NINDS is one of the National Institutes of Health and is dedicated to biomedical research on disorders of the brain and nervous system. Its Web site contains basic information sheets on virtually any neurological disorder as well as more detailed papers on many of them.

National Pain Foundation: www.painconnection.org

The National Pain Foundation, a nonprofit 501(c)(3) organization, was established to advance functional recovery of persons in pain through information, education, and support. Through its Web site, the NPF provides a virtual community for pain patients, their families, and their friends. Information and resources are presented in an interactive way that encourages patients to take an active role in the management of their chronic pain.

3511 S. Clarkson Street
Englewood, CO 80113

The New England Center for Headache (NECH):
www.headachenech.com

The NECH is one of the leading headache and Migraine clinics. Its Web site offers good basic information on different types of headaches and Migraine, rotating "Frequently Asked Questions," rotating "Headache Pearls," and more. There's also the standard information about the clinic and staff.

778 Long Ridge Road
Stamford, CT 06092
Phone: 203-968-8303

Ohio Valley Eye Physicians: www.ohiovalleyeye.com

Ohio Valley Eye Physicians is a group ophthalmology practice in Parkersburg, West Virginia (my hometown!). Not only are these doctors great, but they have a Web site that has great information about eye diseases.

O.U.C.H., Organization for Understanding Cluster Headaches:
www.clusterheadaches.org

The Organization for Understanding Cluster Headaches (O.U.C.H.) is a 501(c)(3) nonprofit organization, formed to assist cluster headache sufferers and their families (supporters). The O.U.C.H. Web site is a great resource for cluster headache sufferers. It has a lot of great information, doctor recommendations, and much more.

The World Headache Alliance (WHA): www.w-h-a.org

The World Headache Alliance (WHA) exists to relieve the suffering of people affected by headache throughout the world, in particular by sharing information among headache organizations and by increasing the awareness and understanding of headache as a public health concern with profound social and economic impact. Its Web site has a great deal of information on headaches and Migraine disease as well as information to help people locate organizations where they live.

3288 Old Coach Road
Burlington, Ontario
CANADA
L7N 3P7

Online Support

Forums (discussion boards)
- ACHE: www.achenet.org/forums/inter.php
- About Headaches and Migraine: www.headaches.about.com/mpboards.htm
- All Info About Headaches and Migraine: www.headaches.allinfoabout.com, click forum button on left
- Help for Headaches and Migraine: helpforheadaches.com/forum/

Yahoo! groups (discussion groups/mailing lists)
- Migraine: health.groups.yahoo.com/group/migraine
- Migraine Help: health.groups.yahoo.com/group/migrainehelp
- The Cluster Buster (cluster headaches) health.groups.yahoo.com/group/TheClusterBusters/

Live online chat room:
- Help for Headaches and Migraine: helpforheadaches.com/chat.htm

U.S. Government Sites for Information

Health and Human Services Office of Civil Rights:
www.hhs.gov/ocr/hipaa/.
HIPAA information.

Medline Plus Headache Topic Index:
www.nlm.nih.gov/medlineplus/headache.html.
From the National Library of Medicine and National Institutes of Health.

Medline Plus Medical Dictionary:
www.nlm.nih.gov/medlineplus/mplusdictionary.html.
Look up medical terms online in the *Merriam-Webster Medical Dictionary*. From the National Library of Medicine and National Institutes of Health.

Medline Plus Medications Information:
www.nlm.nih.gov/medlineplus/druginformation.html.

From the National Library of Medicine and National Institutes of Health, this site offers fairly extensive information on medications.

Medline Plus Migraine Disease Topic Index:
www.nlm.nih.gov/medlineplus/migraine.html.
From the National Library of Medicine and National Institutes of Health.

The National Institute of Neurological Disorders and Stroke (NINDS): www.ninds.nih.gov.

Pharmaceutical Company Sites with Good Educational Content

AstraZeneca, manufacturer of Zomig, www.zomigconsumer.com

GlaxoSmithKline, manufacturer of Imitrex: www.migrainehelp.com

Merck, manufacturer of Maxalt: www.maxalt.com

Ortho-McNeil Pharmaceutical, manufacturer of Axert: www.axert.com

Ortho-McNeil Pharmaceutical, manufacturer of Topamax: www.4migraineprevention.com

Pfizer, manufacturer of Relpax: www.knockoutmigraines.com
This site also offers an exemplary "Understanding in a Box" educational kit to help educate family and friends. It includes a wonderful book for explaining Migraine to children, *Mama Lion's Migraine*.

Advocacy Organizations

National Patient Advocate Foundation: www.npaf.org
The National Patient Advocate Foundation seeks to create avenues of access to insurance funding for evolving therapies, therapeutic devices, and agents through legislative and policy reform.
725 15th Street, NW, Suite 503
Washington, D.C. 20005
Phone: 202-347-8009

Patient Advocate Foundation: www.patientadvocate.org

The Patient Advocate Foundation is a national nonprofit organization that serves as an active liaison between the patient and his or her insurer, employer, and/or creditors to resolve insurance, job retention, and/or debt crisis matters relative to their diagnosis through case managers, doctors, and attorneys. The Patient Advocate Foundation seeks to safeguard patients through effective mediation assuring access to care, maintenance of employment, and preservation of their financial stability.

700 Thimble Shoals Boulevard, Suite 200
Newport News, VA 23606

Patients Are Powerful: www.patientsarepowerful.org

Patients Are Powerful is a diverse nonprofit group of "managed care experts" singularly dedicated to helping patients improve their managed medical health care.

P.O. Box 345
Penryn, CA 95663

Society for Healthcare Consumer Advocacy (SHCA):
www.shca-aha.org/shca-aha/index.jsp

The SHCA is a nonprofit health care organization dedicated to individuals interested in advocacy as well as patient representatives, guest relations professionals, physicians, nurses, social workers, and others currently employed in hospitals, health maintenance organizations, home health agencies, long-term care facilities, and other health-related organizations.

One North Franklin/31N
Chicago, IL 60606
Phone: 312-422-3851

Aromatherapy Supplies

Nature's Gift Aromatherapy Products: www.naturesgift.com
314 Old Hickory Boulevard East
Madison, TN 37115
Phone: 615-612-4270

Camden-Grey Essential Oils: www.camdengrey.com
  3591 NW 82 Avenue
  Miami, FL 33122
  Phone: 877-232-7662 (orders only)
  Phone: 305-500-9630 (other matters, leave message)

Crystals

Crystal Cure: www.crystal-cure.com
  Amerindea
  P.O. Box 69
  Meadow Bridge, WV 25976
  Phone: 626-301-0242

eBay: www.ebay.com
  It can be tricky to find items on eBay, but I've found these two paths to be good for crystals:
  • Everything Else > Metaphysical > Crystal Healing
  • Collectibles > Rocks, Fossils, Minerals > Mineral Specimens > Crystals

APPENDIX D: RECOMMENDED READING

Aromatherapy for Dummies by Kathi Keville
I'm not always a fan of the "Dummies" books, but this one is a great guide for beginners to aromatherapy. Author Kathi Keville, director of the American Herb Association, deftly sheds light on a wide variety of aromas, their sources, and the aid they are said to offer. Choose the fragrant form that works best for you—candles, incense, oils, potpourri, and more. Keville provides information to make you a smart shopper, including where to get aromatherapy products and how to store them. She covers the wide variety of methods in which you can use aromatherapy to your advantage, including ways to bring the right aroma into your workplace.

Clinical Pharmacology Made Incredibly Easy! Published by Springhouse Publishing
Want to know what receptors, neurons, neurotransmitters, and the like are, how and why they work, and what all of it means in relation to our meds? Better yet, want to be able to understand it? Then this book is for you. Filled with all kinds of wonderful diagrams and margin notes, this book really does make it "incredibly easy!"

Cluster Headaches by Michael Goldstein
Goldstein has done an admirable job of compiling excerpts from the experiences of 217 "ClusterHeads." As someone who suffers from cluster headaches himself, he knows what fellow sufferers and those trying to understand them need to know. Goldstein has constructed his book well and arranged the excerpts into a superb range of topics.

The Crystal Bible: A Definitive Guide to Crystals by Judy Hall
Beautifully illustrated, *The Crystal Bible* offers a comprehensive guide to crystals, their shapes, colors, and applications. With informative descriptions and an easy-to-use format, it is an indispensable practical handbook for crystal lovers and users everywhere—both beginner and expert alike.

The book's directory format and beautiful full-color photos ensure that the crystals are easily identifiable. Descriptions, which accompany each of the crystals, provide all the information on their appearance, worldwide distribution, attributes, actions, and healing properties. All the major and less-known stones currently available are contained inside, including those only recently discovered. A comprehensive index cross-referencing crystals to applications, aliments, and conditions makes this book a vital reference for all crystal users.

A Guided Tour of Hell: Migraine, in the Words of Its Sufferers by Kristine Hatak
Do you have people in your life who haven't a clue what you go through with Migraine? If so, this is the book for you! Here is a compilation of Migraineurs' descriptions of Migraine attacks and the effects on their lives. You'll read it and think, "That's me!" Even reading a few pages will have a great impact on any reader.

Headache in Primary Care by Stephen D. Silberstein, Richard B. Lipton, Peter J. Goadsby, Robert T. Smith
Written from the viewpoint of the family doctor, this book is fairly technical, but I found it not to be too technical to understand. Very well organized with excellent charts and illustrations. Deals with all kinds of headache disorders, their diagnosis, the appropriate medications, and so on, with great explanations of the physiology of the headache or attack, how the drugs work, and more. Written by top experts in the field.

Headache Help by Lawrence Robbins, Susan S. Lang; second edition
Describes the wide range of treatments available for migraine, cluster headaches, and tension-type headaches. Excellent, clear information on the actions and side effects of the drugs used to prevent and abort episodes or treat the pain. Includes info on alternative therapies and self-help strategies. Dr. Robbins is an acknowledged expert in the field and a headache/Migraine sufferer himself.

The Headache Prevention Cookbook by David Marks, M.D.; recipes
by Laura Marks, M.D.
Using anecdotes from his own practice, Marks explains which ingredients can cause headaches. He also outlines a way to identify our own
triggers. The potential triggers include a wide list of ordinary foods,
such as beans, chili peppers, dried fruits, canned soup, certain cheeses,
certain vinegars, nuts, chocolate, and ice cream. To help people with
undiagnosed food sensitivities steer clear of the headache-causing cul-
prits, Laura Marks, a doctor and an accomplished cook, has created
more than one hundred easy-to-prepare recipes, including Roast Garlic
Linguine, Lemon-Glazed Chicken, Jewish-Style Baby Artichokes, and
Moist Orange Pound Cake. I've tried some of these recipes. They're
wonderful and easy.

*Living Well with Chronic Fatigue Syndrome and Fibromyalgia:
What Your Doctor Doesn't Tell You That You Need to Know* by Mary
J. Shomon
Many Migraineurs also have chronic fatigue syndrome or fibromyalgia,
so this book my well be of interest to you. A comprehensive guide to
the diagnosis and treatment of chronic fatigue syndrome and
fibromyalgia—vital help for the millions of people suffering from pain,
fatigue, and sleep problems. An estimated 6 million Americans suffer
from fibromyalgia, and eight hundred thousand have chronic fatigue
syndrome. Both conditions are characterized by severe and widespread
pain, debilitating fatigue, and difficulty with concentration and memory. Getting diagnosed can be particularly difficult, and patients must
then navigate conflicting information and the latest fads in order to
choose from among dozens of treatment options. In her trademark accessible, easy-to-follow style, patient advocate Mary J. Shomon ex-
plores these often confusing conditions, highlighting the pros and cons
of conventional and alternative approaches, giving you tips for developing a recovery plan, and providing clear direction and solutions for sufferers of chronic fatigue syndrome and fibromyalgia.

The MemoryMinder Personal Health Journal by MemoryMinder
Journals, Inc.
I quite often emphasize the importance of maintaining a headache and
Migraine diary. However, there are times when we'd like to keep more
information than can be conveniently recorded on the type of diary
page that is simple for our doctors to review and analyze. I was using a

blank journal for that purpose until I came across *The MemoryMinder Personal Health Journal.*

Migraine and Other Headaches by William B. Young and Stephen D. Silberstein

Migraine and Other Headaches is the essential guide for everyone who suffers from headaches and will provide the information needed to obtain effective medical care and long-term relief. Different types of headache are thoroughly explained in easy-to-understand language, beginning with Migraine, the most common severe headache, which occurs in approximately 12 percent of the U.S. population. Also discussed are rebound headache, tension-type headache—the most common primary headache disorder—cluster headache, unusual headaches, nonheadache illnesses that frequently accompany headache, sinus headache, disorders of the neck, post-traumatic headache, and atypical facial pain and trigeminal neuralgia.

The Thyroid Diet: Manage Your Metabolism for Lasting Weight Loss by Mary J. Shomon

Thyroid disease also seems to be very common among Migraineurs, so many of you will undoubtedly find this book useful. From patient advocate Mary Shomon, author of the best-selling *Living Well with Hypothyroidism,* comes *The Thyroid Diet*—the first book to tackle the critical connection between weight gain and thyroid disease, offering a conventional and alternative plan for lasting weight loss. More than 25 million Americans have diagnosed—and undiagnosed—thyroid conditions, which almost always result in a metabolic slowdown. *The Thyroid Diet* helps many previously unsuccessful dieters get diagnosed and treated—and proper thyroid treatment may be all that's needed to lose weight successfully. Even after optimal treatment, however, weight problems plague many thyroid patients. For those patients, *The Thyroid Diet* identifies the many frustrating impediments to weight loss and offers solutions—both conventional and alternative—to help.

Understanding Migraine and Other Headaches by Stewart J. Tepper

Understanding Migraine and Other Headaches provides up-to-date information on the causes and diagnoses as well as current preventive measures, effective treatments, and surgical procedures. This overview includes discussion of every major type of headache, including the debilitating, nausea-inducing forms of Migraine, episodic tension-type headaches (the most common form), chronic daily headaches, and more obscure headaches such as trigeminal neuralgia and cluster headaches. This book undertakes a comprehensive look at medications for acute "as needed" treatment of headaches and for preventing the onset of an attack. It offers guidelines for assessing headache pain, the level and type of medication needed, possible side effects, and drug effectiveness.

You Are Not Your Illness: Seven Principles for Meeting the Challenge by Linda Noble Topf, M.A., with Hal Zina Bennett, Ph.D.

We all know how Migraine disease and chronic headaches can tend to take over our lives. We have to be careful or we think of our lives in terms of our illness. Topf, who has lived most of her adulthood with multiple sclerosis, offers us not platitudes, but actual principles for meeting the challenges of everyday life. There's a great deal of wisdom in this book. Don't expect it to be a simple read, but it's absolutely worth reading.

APPENDIX E: REFERENCED EXPERTS

Jan Lewis Brandes, M.D., is a headache and Migraine specialist practicing in Nashville, Tennessee. She was a Fulbright scholar and earned her medical degree at Vanderbilt University of Medicine. Dr. Brandes is a Fellow of the American Headache Society and a national lecturer and has published many research papers. She has also been very actively involved in clinical trials of medications.

300 20th Avenue North, Suite 603
Nashville, TN 37203
Phone: 615-284-4680

Michael John Coleman is co-founder and executive director of MAGNUM, the National Migraine Association. Michael John has suffered from intractable Migraines since the age of six and has experienced the life-altering effects of the disease firsthand. MAGNUM's use of art and media in its public awareness efforts allows Michael John to divide his time between Migraine disease awareness advocacy and his fine-art career. The union of his talents was noted in the October 2001 *WHA Rome, Italy, Abridged Migraine Disease Awareness Art Exhibition,* a solo exhibit in (of course) Rome, Italy, featuring his landscapes and figure studies, including his June 2001 New York City cityscapes and post-9/11 *Angel Flag* series. In addition, he continued to blend his art with his medical advocacy when he lectured about *Migraines and Art* in Sicily, Italy, and again on this issue in Istanbul, Turkey, for the European Headache Society. He represented American headache non-governmental organizations at the World Health Organization headquarters in Geneva, Switzerland, in 2000 for the first ever *Meeting on Headache and Related Disorders.* Michael John hand-carried the first policy letter from a White House recognizing Migraine disease as a major public health issue in 2001. Thanks to his efforts, President George

W. Bush became the first American president to acknowledge the burden of Migraine. Michael John also hand-carried a letter from Secretary of Health and Human Services Tommy Thompson to the Rome Headache Congress in 2003, another first. He worked with MAGNUM's co-founder Ms. Terri Miller Burchfield to create the world's most popular Migraine Web site, www.migraines.org, in 1996. Michael and Terri have presented or lectured on Migraine disease awareness from the Agency of Healthcare Policy and Research to the CDC National Center for Health Statistics. Michael John has advanced his advocacy work from national print media and the Internet to radio and TV, including ABC, NBC, CBS, FOXNews, CNN, PBS, VOA, and MSNBC, to name a few. He has worked with the author on many projects over the years to facilitate a better understanding of Migraine disease and headache disorders. To learn more about Michael John's health advocacy work, you can visit www.migraines.org; you can also access www.MichaelJohnColeman.com to learn about his artwork.

Steven Halpern, Ph.D., began his pioneering research exploring sound, consciousness, and healing using brain wave biofeedback and Kirlian (aura) photography. He is the author of *Sound Health* (Harper & Row, 1985), numerous articles, and a syndicated monthly newsletter. Dr. Halpern is the world's leading composer and recording artist of music for relaxation, wellness, and "sound health." For over thirty years, he has pioneered and promoted the healing powers of music through his recordings, books, media appearances, and workshops. His unique use of musical tone, time, and space has helped millions to enjoy the stillness and peaceful place that lies within each of us. His music resonates in the key of the heart and strikes a chord that we recognize and appreciate intuitively. The free-floating ambience and luminous sound quality make it easy to heed the advice of spiritual teachers throughout the ages: "Be still . . . and know."

Learn more about Dr. Halpern's work at www.stevenhalpern.com.

John Claude Krusz, M.D., Ph.D., received his Ph.D. in neuropharmacology from the State University of New York, Downstate Medical Center, in 1975 and his medical degree from the State University of New York at Buffalo School of Medicine in 1983. He is a diplomate of the American Board of Neurology and Psychiatry and the American Board of Forensic Examiners. He is board certified in pain management, EEG, and quantitative electroencephalography. He is the vice president of the American Board of Electroencephalography and Neurophysiology. Dr. Krusz currently serves on the editorial board of the American Academy of Pain Management and is an adjunct faculty member in the Department of Psychology at Southern Methodist University. Dr. Krusz has been involved in extensive research in the area of headache and pain disorders. He is in private practice in neurology in Dallas and serves as the head of his multidisciplinary clinic, Anodyne Headache and PainCare. Dr. Krusz's primary areas of interest include evaluation and novel treatments of headaches, pain syndromes, and neurobehavioral disorders. He is especially interested in outpatient treatment issues, especially where intravenous acute management of symptoms is concerned. Neuropsychiatric interests include traumatic brain injury, Tourette's syndrome, Asperger's syndrome, attention deficit disorders, and deaf- and hard-of-hearing-related problems. He helped found the National Deaf People's Institute in Dallas.

ANODYNE Headache and PainCare
5446 Glen Lakes Drive
Dallas, TX 75231
Phone: 214-750-6664

Richard B. Lipton, M.D., is professor and vice chairman of neurology and professor of epidemiology and population health at the Albert Einstein College of Medicine in New York. He is also the Lotti and Bernard Benson Faculty Scholar at the Albert Einstein College of Medicine and director of the Montefiore Headache Unit. Dr. Lipton holds leadership positions in several professional societies. He is a past president of the American Headache Society and on the Executive Committee of the International Headache Society. He is an associate editor of both _Cephalalgia_ and _Headache_ and on the editorial boards of several journals, including _Neurology._ Dr. Lipton has made numerous contributions to the neurology literature. He has published more than four hundred original articles and reviews, as well as six books. His interests include headache epidemiology and clinical trials, cognitive aging, and dementia as well as outcomes research. He has twice received the H. G. Wolff Research Award from the American Headache Society and is the recipient (with Peter J. Goadsby, M.D., and Stephen Silberstein, M.D.) of the Medical Book Award from the British Medical Association for his text _Headache in Clinical Practice_ (1998). He is coeditor (with Stephen Silberstein, M.D., and Donald Dalessio, M.D.) of _Wolff's Headache and Other Head Pain_ (7th ed.).

Montefiore Headache Unit
3326 Rochambeau Avenue
Bronx, NY 10467
Phone: 718-920-4636

Fred Sheftell, M.D., is the founder and director of the New England Center for Headache in Stamford, Connecticut. He is also a well-known researcher and author in the field. He is past president of the American Council of Education, and medical adviser chairman of MAGNUM, the National Migraine Association; he has lectured widely throughout the world and been a guest on NPR's *Fresh Air* and numerous other national television shows. He is a recipient of the United Way's Silver Award and the American Council for Headache Education's Lifetime Achievement Award. He is listed in Woodward and White's *Best Doctors in America.*

New England Center for Headache
788 Long Ridge Road
Stamford, CT 06902
Phone: 203-968-1799

Suzanne E. Simons, executive director, has provided leadership to the National Headache Foundation, a nonprofit organization dedicated to serving headache sufferers and their health care providers, for eighteen years. She is a respected authority on the public concerns of headache and head pain. She served on the Institutional Review Board for Protection of Human Subjects Committee for the Rosalind Franklin University of Medicine and Science, formerly FUHS/Chicago Medical School, from 1992 to 2004. She was a member of the Primary Headache Project of the Foundation for Accountability, an expert panel developing standardized measurements for use in the health care field. Ms. Simons served on the editorial board of *The Brain Matters*, a special supplement to *USA Today.* Her own headache-related articles have been published in the American Pain Society's *Bulletin* and the Ohio Society of Office Nursing's *Office Call.* She was previously a member of the boards of directors of the National Society of Fund Raising Executives and the Kent State University Alumni Association.

Melissa C. Stöppler, M.D., is a physician, researcher, and writer with an interest in stress and its effects on the human body. A board-certified anatomic pathologist, Dr. Stöppler has held medical school faculty positions at Georgetown University and the University of Marburg, Germany. Dr. Stöppler's educational background includes a B.A. from the University of Virginia and an M.D. from the University of North Carolina. Currently, she is editor and producer and Guide of the stress management site on the About.com network:www.stress.about.com.

Scott H. Strickler, M.D., attended medical school at West Virginia University College of Medicine, where he was vice president of Alpha Omega Alpha, an organization reserved for those in the top 10 percent of their medical school class. He completed his internship at Riverside Hospital in Columbus, Ohio. He received his ophthalmology training at the Ohio State University College of Medicine. Dr. Strickler is board certified by the American Board of Ophthalmology. He is a fellow of the American Academy of Ophthalmology and a member of the American Society of Cataract and Refractive Surgery. Dr. Strickler's special interests include topical cataract surgery and glaucoma and diabetic eye care.

Ohio Valley Eye Physicians
416 Grand Park Drive
Parkersburg, WV 26101
Phone: 304-428-3500
www.OhioValleyEye.com

Stewart Tepper, M.D., received his undergraduate degree cum laude from Yale University and his medical degree from Cornell University Medical College. He completed his residency in neurology at Harvard Medical School, Boston. Dr. Tepper is director of the New England Center for Headache and of the New England Research Institute in Stamford, Connecticut, and is assistant clinical professor of Neurology at Yale University Medical School. He has authored over 150 professional papers and 7 books, most recently *Understanding Migraine and Other Headaches* (University of Mississippi Press, 2004). His interests in teaching and patient care have led him to his current positions on the Education Committee of the American Headache Society, the Education and Membership Committee of the International Headache Society, and the board of directors of the American Council on Headache Education and of the Headache Cooperative of New England.

New England Center for Headache
788 Long Ridge Road
Stamford, CT 06902
Phone: 203-968-1799

William B. Young, M.D., is associate professor of neurology and director of the in-patient program at the Jefferson Headache Center at Thomas Jefferson University. He is an active member of the American Academy of Neurology and a Fellow of the American Headache Society. He is peer reviewer for *Headache: The Journal of Head and Face Pain* and *Cephalalgia.* Dr Young was recently awarded the American Association for the Study of Headache/Eli Lilly Headache and Depression Research Award to study the major influence of major depression on outcomes in transformed Migraine. He is involved in many ongoing research projects on Migraine and cluster headache.

Jefferson Headache Center
8130 Gibbon Building
111 South 11th Street
Philadelphia, PA 19107
Phone: 215-955-2243

APPENDIX F: REFERENCES

Chapter 1

World Health Organization. "Headache Disorders." The World Health Organization Media Center, Fact Sheet No. 277. March 2004. Accessible at www.who.int/mediacentre/factsheets/fs277/en/.

Hu X. Henry, Leona E. Markson, Richard B. Lipton, Walter F. Stewart, and Marc L. Berger. "Burden of Migraine in the United States: Disability and Economic Costs." *Archives of Internal Medicine* 159, no. 8 (1999): 813–818.

National Statistics Online. United Kingdom Census Data, www.statistics.gov.uk.

Statistics Canada. Population by Sex and Age Group. Accessible at www.statcan.ca/english/Pgdb/demo10a.htm.

The Pharmaceutical Research and Manufacturers of America. "Productivity Impact Model." Accessible at www.migrainecalculator.com.

Dowson A., C. Dahlof, S. Tepper, and L. Newman. "Prevalence and Diagnosis of Migraine in a Primary Care Setting." Abstract PA.30, presented at the 14th Migraine Trust International Symposium, September 24, 2002. London.

Discovery Health Channel. "Headache Timeline." Accessible at health.discovery.com/centers/headaches/timeline/timeline.html.

Pain Management Technologies. "Early Developments in Electroanalgesia: In the Beginning." Accessible at www.paintechnology.com/051.htm.

Silberstein, Stephen D., M.D., Alan Stiles, D.M.D., William B. Young, M.D., and Todd D. Rozen, M.D. *An Atlas of Headache*. New York: Parthenon Publishing Group, 2002.

Chapter 4

The International Headache Society. "The International Classification of Headache Disorders," 2nd ed. *Cephalalgia* 24, supp. 2 (2004).

Robbins, Lawrence, M.D., and Susan S. Lang. *Headache Help*. Boston: Houghton Mifflin Company, 2000.

Silberstein, Stephen D., Richard B. Lipton, Peter J. Goadsby, and Robert T. Smith. *Headache in Primary Care*. Oxford, UK: Isis Medical Media Ltd., 1999.

World Health Organization. "Headache Disorders."

Young, William B., and Stephen D. Silberstein. *Migraine and Other Headaches*. St. Paul, Minn.: AAN Press, 2004.

Chapter 5

The International Headache Society. "International Classification of Headache Disorders."

Cheyette, Sarah, M.D. *MOMMY, My Head Hurts*. New York: Newmarket Press, 2001.

Robbins and Lang. *Headache Help*.

Silberstein, Stephen D., Richard B. Lipton, and Peter J. Goadsby. *Headache in Clinical Practice*, 2nd ed. Florence, Ky.: Taylor & Francis Group, 2002.

Silberstein et al. *Headache in Primary Care*.

Tepper, Stewart J., M.D. *Understanding Migraine and Other Headaches*. Jackson, Miss.: University of Mississippi Press, 2004.

Young and Silberstein. *Migraine and Other Headaches*.

Etminan, Mahar, Bahi Takkouche, Francisco Caamaño Isorna, and Ali Samii. "Risk of Ischaemic Stroke in People with Migraine: Systematic Review and Meta-analysis of Observational Studies." *British Medical Journal* 330 (January 8, 2005):63–65.

Coleman, Michael John. "Dancing with Migraine as a Youth." MAGNUM, the National Migraine Association, www.migraines.org.

Chapter 6

Goldstein, Michael. *Cluster Headaches*. Santa Fe, N.M.: New Atlantean Press, 1999.

The International Headache Society. "International Classification of Headache Disorders."

Silberstein et al. *Headache in Clinical Practice.*

Silberstein et al. *Headache in Primary Care.*

Silberstein, Stephen D., M.D., Richard B. Lipton, M.D., and Donald J. Dalessio, M.D. *Wolff's Headache and Other Head Pain,* 7th ed. New York: Oxford University Press, 2001.

Young and Silberstein. *Migraine and Other Headaches.*

Chapter 7

"A Profile of U.S. Poison Centers in 2001: A Survey Conducted by the American Association of Poison Control Centers." American Association of Poison Control Centers. Washington, D.C.

Loder, Elizabeth, and David Biondi. "Oral Phenobarbital Loading: A Safe and Effective Method of Withdrawing Patients with Headache from Butalbital Compounds." *Headache: The Journal of Head and Face Pain* 43, no. 8 (2003):904–09.

Robbins and Lang. *Headache Help.*

Saper, Joel R., M.D., Stephen Silberstein, M.D., C. David Gordon, M.D., Robert L. Hamel, P.A.-C., and Sahar Swidan, Pharm.D. *Handbook of Headache Management.* Baltimore, Md.: Lippincott Williams & Wilkins, 1999.

Silberstein et al. *Headache in Primary Care.*

"Teenager Accidentally Overdoses on Over-the-Counter Analgesic." Associated Press. July 2, 2003. Accessible at ChannelOklahoma.com.

Tepper, Stewart J., M.D., Fred D. Sheftell, M.D., and Alan M. Rapoport, M.D., eds. *The Spectrum of Migraine.* New York: McMahon Publishing Group, 2002.

Chapter 8

Newman, Lawrence C., M.D. "Effective Management of Ice Pick Pains, SUNCT, and Episodic and Chronic Paroxysmal Hemicrania." *Current Pain and Headache Reports* 5(2001):292–99.

Rozen, Todd D., M.D. "Short-Lasting Headache Syndromes and Treatment Options." *Current Pain and Headache Reports* 8(2004):268–73.

Tepper. *Understanding Migraine and Other Headaches.*

Young and Silberstein. *Migraine and Other Headaches.*

Saper et al. *Handbook of Headache Management,* 241–42.

Evans, Randolph W., and R. Couch. "Orgasm and Migraine." *Headache: The Journal of Head and Face Pain* 111, no. 6 (2001):512–14.

Chapter 11

Robins and Lang. *Headache Help.*

Halpern, Steven. *Effortless Relaxation.* CD. San Anselmo, Calif.: Inner Peace Music, 1991.

Saper et al. *Handbook of Headache Management.*

Chapter 12

Young and Silberstein. *Migraine and Other Headaches.*

Ramadan, Nahib M., M.D., Stephen D. Silberstein, M.D., F.A.C.P., Frederick G. Freitag, D.O., Thomas T. Gilbert, M.D., M.P.H., and Benjamin M. Fishbert, M.D. "Evidence-Based Guidelines for Migraine Headache in the Primary Care Setting: Pharmacological Management for Prevention of Migraine." *American Academy of Neurology* (2000).

Lewis, D., M.D., S. Ashwal, M.D., A. Hershey, M.D., D. Hirtz, M.D., M. Yonker, M.D., and S. Silberstein, M.D. "Pharmacological Treatment of Migraine Headache in Children and Adolescents." *Neurology* 63 (2004): 2215–24.

Silberstein, Stephen D., Ninan Mathew, Joel Saper, and Stephen Jenkins. "Botulinum Toxin Type A as a Migraine Preventive Treatment." *Headache: The Journal of Head and Face Pain* 40, no. 6 (2000):445–50.

Rozen, T. D., M. L. Oshinsky, C. A. Gebeline, K. C. Bradley, W. B. Young, A. L. Shechter, and S. D. Silberstein. "Open Label Trial of Coenzyme Q10 as a Migraine Preventive." *Cephalalgia* 22, no. 2 (2002):37–41.

Chapter 13

Baronov, David, Ph.D. *Everything You Need to Know About Feverfew and Migraines.* New York: Prima Health, 1999.

Dodick, David, Richard B. Lipton, Vincent Martin, Vasilios Papademetriou, Wayne Rosamond, Antoinette MaassenVanDenBrink, Hassan Loutfi, K. Michael Welch, Peter J. Goadsby, Steven Hahn, Susan Hutchinson, David Matchar, Stephen Silberstein, Timothy R. Smith, R. Allan Purdy, and Jane Saiers. "Consensus Statement: Cardiovascular Safety Profile of Triptans (5-HT1B/1D Agonists) in the Acute Treatment of Migraine." *Headache: The Journal of Head and Face Pain* 44, no. 5 (2004):414–25.

Chapter 15

Baronov, David, Ph.D. *Everything You Need to Know About Feverfew and Migraines*. New York: Prima Health, 1999.

Biofeedback Certification Institute of America. Accessible at www.bcia.org.

Biofeedback Infocenter. Accessible at www.holistic-online.com/Biofeedback.htm.

National Center for Complementary and Alternative Medicine. "What Is Acupuncture." About Holistic Healing, healing.about.com/od/acupuncture/ss/whatisacpunctre.htm.

Young and Silberstein. *Migraine and Other Headaches*.

Vickers, A. J., R. W. Rees, C. E. Zollman, R. McCarney, C. M. Smith, et al. "Acupuncture for Chronic Headache in Primary Care: Large, Pragmatic, Randomised Trial." *British Medical Journal* 328, no. 7442(2004):747.

Chapter 17

Carter, Alden R. *Mama Lion's Migraine*. New York: Pfizer, Inc. 2004

Chapter 20

104th Congress. Public Law 104-191. "Health Insurance Portability and Accountability Act of 1996 (HIPAA)." United States Department of Health and Human Services, Office for Civil Rights, www.hhs.gov/ocr/hipaa.

Chapter 23

Sorgen, Carol. "To Stay Healthy . . . Make Friends," Medscape Health for Consumers. December 2001. Accessible at health.medscape.com/viewarticle/411465.

INDEX

WANT TO LIVE WELL?

LIVING WELL WITH MIGRAINE DISEASE AND HEADACHES
What Your Doctor Doesn't Tell You . . . That You Need to Know
by Teri Robert
0-06-076685-9 (trade paperback)
A holistic, patient-centered guide to the diagnosis, side effects and treatments for headaches and Migraine disease.

LIVING WELL WITH MENOPAUSE
What Your Doctor Doesn't Tell You . . . That You Need To Know
by Carolyn Chambers Clark, ARNP, Ed.D.
0-06-075812-0 (trade paperback)
A complete holistic guide and self-care manual to menopause.

LIVING WELL WITH HYPOTHYROIDISM
What Your Doctor Doesn't Tell You . . . That You Need to Know
by Mary J. Shomon
0-06-074095-7 (trade paperback)
An expanded and updated edition of the hugely successful *Living Well with Hypothyroidism.*

LIVING WELL WITH GRAVES' DISEASE AND HYPERTHYROIDISM
What Your Doctor Doesn't Tell You . . . That You Need to Know
by Mary J. Shomon
0-06-073019-6 (trade paperback)
Here is a holistic road map for diagnosis, treatment, and recovery from Graves' disease and hyperthyroidism.

LIVING WELL WITH EPILEPSY AND OTHER SEIZURE DISORDERS
An Expert Explains What You Really Need to Know
by Carl W. Bazil. M.D., Ph.D
0-06-053848-1 (trade paperback)
A much-needed book of information, support, and lifestyle strategies for this surprisingly common problem.

LIVING WELL WITH ENDOMETRIOSIS
What Your Doctor Doesn't Tell You . . . That You Need to Know
by Kerry-Ann Morris
0-06-084426-4 (trade paperback)
A complete guide to the side effects and treatments—both conventional and alternative—for endometriosis.

LIVING WELL WITH CHRONIC FATIGUE SYNDROME AND FIBROMYALGIA
What Your Doctor Doesn't Tell You . . . That You Need to Know
by Mary J. Shomon
0-06-052125-2 (trade paperback)
A comprehensive guide to the diagnosis and treatment of chronic fatigue syndrome and fibromyalgia.

LIVING WELL WITH AUTOIMMUNE DISEASE
What Your Doctor Doesn't Tell You . . . That You Need to Know
by Mary J. Shomon
0-06-093819-6 (trade paperback)
A complete guide to understanding the mysterious disorders of the immune system.

LIVING WELL WITH ANXIETY
What Your Doctor Doesn't Tell You . . . That You Need to Know
by Carolyn Chambers Clark, ARNP, Ed.D.
0-06-082377-1 (trade paperback)
A complete guide to the side effects and treatments for anxiety disorders.

Visit www.AuthorTracker.com
for exclusive information on your favorite HarperCollins authors.

Available wherever books are sold, or call 1-800-331-3761 to order.